READ THIS IF YOU HAVE A HEART

By Elie Klein, ND

Title: Read This If You Have A Heart

All rights reserved.

© 2013 Dr. Elie Klein, BSc, ND

978-1927677537

Contents

ACKNOWLEDGEMENTS

Many people and factors have been influential, inspirational and helpful in writing this book.

First, I would like to thank, faculty, administrative and clinical staff of the Canadian College of Naturopathic Medicine for providing me a strong foundation in naturopathic medicine and medical sciences.

Over the last few decades, many researchers and doctors have done important work in educating the public and bringing to light misconceptions and truths regarding the causes and cures of cardiovascular disease. Their writings have been a great resource to draw upon in guiding my clinical work and the content of my Dr. Klein's Healthy Heart Program™ and, of course, in creating this book. Some of the most influential have been Dr. Joseph Mercola, DO; Dr. Uffe Ravneskov, MD; Dr. Ray Peat, PhD; Dr. Stephan Guyenet, PhD; Dr. Gerry Bohemier; and others.

My patients and my students (of Dr. Klein's Healthy Heart Program™) have inspired me to stay well read and stay on top of current research and writings about various aspects of cardiovascular disease, so I can deliver the care and the education required to help them resolve their health concerns.

I would like to thank my editor Wendy Almeida for her patience and guidance in developing this book.

As well, special thanks to Raymond Aaron and the 10-10-10 crew who inspired me and guided me in taking a stalled, unfinished book and making it a published reality in a few short months.

Special thanks to my parents for their life-time support, including their support during my naturopathic medical education, and to my kids Sarah, Yael and David, who offer so much love and vitality. Last, but not least, to my loving wife, who patiently encouraged me for years to write this book and who was practically a co-creator of this book. I love and appreciate you all.

FOREWORD

In this book, Dr. Elie Klein provides revolutionary, yet incredibly simple, solutions to the world's number one cause of death, cardiovascular disease and its associated risk factors. After having read this book, it became obvious to me that following the standard dietary recommendations of limiting the dietary intake of saturated fat, cholesterol and salt as a means of dealing with heart disease, has done nothing to reverse this worldwide pandemic. Focusing on these dietary guidelines has been nothing but a diversion from the real causes of cardiovascular disease. Dr. Klein demonstrates that so many people have been afflicted unnecessarily by heart attacks and strokes because the dietary advice that has been disseminated over the last several decades by doctors and public health agencies has been false. In this book, Dr. Klein provides compelling scientific evidence to support this idea. He also sheds a brilliant light on the true dietary causes of cardiovascular disease, and supports his views with scientific evidence as well as with clear, simple-to-understand explanations.

Read This If You Have a Heart will provide you with the knowledge you need to lower your blood pressure, to ensure healthy cholesterol levels, to improve your blood sugar levels, and, most importantly, to prevent and reverse arterial plaque in order to prevent the occurrence of a heart attack or a stroke.

This book has been so enlightening to read; I learned so much, as will you.

For example, you will learn to recognize the potential harmful effects of pharmaceutical drugs for high blood pressure and cholesterol. These drugs are designed to address only the symptoms, they don't actually treat the cause of cardiovascular disease. You will understand the true causes of cardiovascular disease and what foods and vitamins can help you successfully treat ninety percent of cardiovascular disease.

So many people succumb to a cardiac event or stroke with no pre-existing warning signs. This book will teach you how to recognize potential signs and symptoms of plaque in the arteries, in order to help you determine whether you are at risk.

As Dr. Klein explains in this book, since the dietary causes of cardiovascular disease and its risk factors often contribute to other health problems, such as diabetes, obesity, arthritis, gastro-intestinal issues and so on, by implementing the suggestions provided in the book, you can expect improvements in these conditions as well.

This book offers so much hope and makes it obvious that it is possible to eradicate cardiovascular disease, an unnecessary world-wide pandemic, and save many lives as a result of that.

Raymond Aaron

New York Times best seller co-author of *Chicken Soup for the Parent's Soul* and author of *Chicken Soup for the Canadian Soul*.

INTRODUCTION

Congratulations on picking up *Read This If You Have a Heart*. As outrageous as it may sound, by the time you finish reading this book, you will likely know more than most doctors about how to prevent and reverse the leading cause of death in the world, cardiovascular disease, without drugs.

Doctors and public health agencies tell us that we can prevent heart disease by limiting the intake of saturated fat, dietary cholesterol and salt. Indeed, for several decades now, North Americans have been eating considerably less saturated fat and dietary cholesterol, while salt levels have remained stable.[1,2] Unfortunately, these recommendations have failed us. US government statistics reveal that every year more and more people experience heart attacks, strokes and high blood pressure,[3,4] as well as other related conditions such as obesity and diabetes[5].

My interest in the prevention and in the safe and effective treatment of cardiovascular disease began when I started my naturopathic practice about ten years ago. I was getting a disproportionately high number of patients with risk factors for cardiovascular disease: high blood pressure, high cholesterol, diabetes and other related conditions. They all told me that they were doing the "right thing". They were limiting their intake of fat, cholesterol and salt. Most of them didn't smoke, either. Yet despite these measures, their health failed, and they ended up on multiple medications for blood pressure, cholesterol and diabetes.

In my naturopathic medical training I learned from the same text books that conventional medical students learned from, and I, too, once thought that prevention of cardiovascular disease depended, amongst other factors, on limiting saturated fat, cholesterol and salt.

There is a saying that the definition of insanity is doing the same thing over and over again and expecting different results. Obviously, the conventional wisdom on preventing cardiovascular disease wasn't working.

My curiosity got the best of me. I needed to find out why the current recommendations were not working and what the true causes of cardiac disease were. So for the past decade, I have researched extensively the various causes and various treatment choices of cardiovascular disease.

I came across mountains of scientific information that contradicted the current "wisdom" that saturated fats, cholesterol and salt cause cardiovascular disease.

To summarize the research, it turns out that many of the foods we typically restrict in attempting to prevent heart disease are actually healthy and important to our well-being. Meanwhile, there are other types of food that we have been erroneously eating too much of, which, as it turns out, are the true culprits of cardiovascular disease and diabetes.

You may wonder why doctors and public health officials who are supposed to help protect our health would make recommendations that would be potentially harmful. Unfortunately, it takes time for new paradigms and scientific discoveries to become accepted. While we expect science to be objective, unfortunately, powerful social, commercial and political interests may want to protect old beliefs.

To explain it all in detail would add many more pages to a book that I'd like to keep brief and simple. You can find more about the political and economic influences on the healthcare system in links listed on my website *www.drkleinhealthyheart.com.*

Upon discovering the true causes of high blood pressure and cholesterol, I started making these different yet necessary dietary recommendations to my clients – and witnessed them dramatically improve. Clients who complied experienced improved blood pressure, circulation, cholesterol levels, blood sugar levels and energy levels within weeks. More important, patients with advanced blockages in their coronary arteries were able to reverse these blockages. It has been very gratifying to witness these improvements in my clients, which allowed them to let go of most or all of their medications.

From the knowledge and experience I gained about this topic, I became convinced that it is possible to eradicate ninety percent of all cardiovascular disease (you will understand why ninety percent in the next chapter). This untapped information was revolutionary, yet so simple. It was information that people needed to know in order to avoid becoming statistical casualties of cardiovascular disease, to avert a heart attack or a stroke. There was, however, one limiting factor – time. There was only so much I could teach in half-an-hour to an hour-long patient visit in my office.

The need to adequately educate and mentor people on how to prevent and reverse cardiovascular disease and its risk factors inspired me to write this book and to create a special education and mentoring program called *Dr. Klein's Healthy Heart Program™*. The program is designed to provide the necessary knowledge and guidance, as well as practical tools and exercises, to help clients make truly healthy dietary and lifestyle choices.

This book is a summary of much of what I learned and what I teach my clients and my Healthy Heart Program students. It is a summary of my current understanding and experience to date of what generally needs to be done to reverse risk factors of cardiovascular disease (including diabetes).

Here you will learn which foods you truly need to avoid and which nutrients you should consume in order to prevent cardiovascular disease, to restore your health and, most important, to increase your chances of preventing a heart attack or a stroke altogether.

By the time you finish this book, you will have important fundamental knowledge that will likely allow you to escape the leading cause of death in the world. You will also be in a position to lead a generally healthier – and longer – life.

This book is an educational tool to help empower you with the information you need to make better choices about your health. However, this book does not constitute treatment and does not replace treatment provided by a qualified healthcare provider.

Let's begin!

CHAPTER 1

DEFINING CARDIOVASCULAR DISEASE

The Leading Cause of Death in the World

What do we mean by cardiovascular disease?

Cardiovascular disease, supposedly a preventable disease, is the leading cause of death in the world, accounting for over 700,000 deaths annually in the US (combined number of deaths from heart disease and stroke)[6], for upwards of 60,000 in Canada[7] and for about 17 million deaths worldwide[8]. However, because it is preventable, this tragedy can be stopped within a few short years once the public learns what the true causes are and implements new dietary and lifestyle habits.

Typically, the term *heart disease* is used inaccurately as a synonym for cardiovascular disease. However, heart disease refers to any disorder that affects the heart, while cardiovascular disease includes both the heart and the blood vessels. For the purpose of this book, I will use the term cardiovascular disease and use the accepted abbreviation CVD.

CVD includes many conditions, such as heart valve disease, arrhythmia, heart failure, orthostatic hypotension, shock, endocarditis and congenital heart disease.

According to the Canadian Heart and Stroke Foundation, over 90% of heart attacks are caused by atherosclerosis! Atherosclerosis is also implicated in half or more of all cases of stroke. This is an important point. If we can figure out how to prevent and reverse atherosclerosis, we will prevent 90% of all heart attacks, at least 50% of all strokes and save hundreds of millions of lives. In fact, I believe that implementing the suggestions laid out in this book will also help prevent more than 90% of all strokes.

What is atherosclerosis?

Atherosclerosis is defined as the hardening of the arteries and narrowing of the arteries from plaque build-up. Arterial plaque consists of white blood cells (immune system cells), fat, cholesterol, calcium, connective tissue and other substances. Plaque build-up disrupts blood flow and reduces delivery of oxygen to different parts of the body. If the coronary arteries (the arteries that surround and nourish the heart) become blocked completely, a heart attack occurs. If plaque blocks the arteries that go to the brain or that are present within the brain, a stroke could occur. Atherosclerosis is what has turned CVD into a worldwide epidemic. It is caused primarily by poor lifestyle and dietary choices.

Currently, according to conventional medicine, high levels of cholesterol in the blood constitute the primary cause of atherosclerosis. However, as you will learn later on in this book, contrary to misguided popular belief, too much cholesterol is NOT the direct cause of plaque in the arteries.

Atherosclerosis and high blood pressure

Most Americans diagnosed with CVD also have chronic high blood pressure, or hypertension.

To me it is pretty clear that atherosclerosis is closely linked to hypertension (a condition of persistent elevated blood pressure). Conventional medicine, however, is more ambiguous about the relationship between atherosclerosis and hypertension.

Medical textbooks identify two forms of hypertension: essential hypertension and secondary hypertension.

Let's start by briefly discussing secondary hypertension. *Secondary hypertension* accounts for only 5% of hypertension cases and results from other pre-existing conditions, such as kidney disease, hormonal disturbances (Cushing's disease, hyperthyroidism, etc.), certain cancers and certain medications. Secondary hypertension is generally not thought of as a condition caused by atherosclerosis, except when atherosclerosis affects the arteries that feed blood and oxygen to the kidneys, a matter that can lead to diminished kidney function.

Essential hypertension, on the other hand, accounts for approximately 95% of all cases and is closely related to atherosclerosis. Although medical textbooks do not identify a direct cause of essential hypertension, many contributing factors are listed. These include smoking, aging, obesity, potassium deficiency, vitamin D deficiency, sedentary lifestyle, salt, alcoholic intake, genetics and stress.

Well, most, if not all of the factors that contribute to essential hypertension also contribute to atherosclerosis, to narrowing of the arteries.

Throughout a person's lifetime, as atherosclerosis sets in, the volume of blood that travels through the arteries remains the same; however, the width of the arteries decreases as they become gradually narrower. As atherosclerosis sets in, the flexibility of the arteries and their ability to contract and relax diminishes. As a result, the pressure the blood exerts against the arteries increases and hypertension develops. Under these circumstances the heart has to work harder pumping the same amount of blood through narrower and stiffer arteries. This increases the strain on the heart and the pressure inside the heart as it pumps the blood into the arteries.

By reversing atherosclerosis, it is then possible to reverse essential hypertension and to reduce the strain on the heart.

The good news is, it is fairly simple to both prevent and reverse atherosclerosis.

Diagnosing high blood pressure

To receive a diagnosis of high blood pressure, or hypertension, your blood pressure must be high on three consecutive blood pressure readings taken on different days.

Blood pressure consists of two numbers. The first number is called *systolic* and its normal range is between 120mmHg to 140 mmHg. This number measures the pressure the heart exerts when it contracts to pump blood to the arteries. The second number is called *diastolic* and its normal range is between 80mmHg to 90mmHg. The diastolic number measures the pressure when the heart is relaxed, in between "pumps".

The difference between the systolic number and the diastolic number is called *pulse* pressure (not to be confused with a *pulse*, which is used to determine a heart rate). Often a pulse pressure that is consistently 50 or more can be indicative of atherosclerosis. To illustrate, someone whose blood pressure is 140/90 has a pulse pressure of 50 (140-90=50), whereas when the blood pressure reading is 120/80, the pulse pressure is 40 (120-80=40).

If you were diagnosed with high blood pressure, your doctor would then attempt to determine if it is essential hypertension or secondary hypertension. If he or she determines that it is essential, then the likely cause is, at least in part, atherosclerosis. In young individuals ongoing stress can also cause hypertension.

You should be aware that some people may get misdiagnosed as having hypertension if their blood pressure shoots up because they get nervous at the doctor's office. This is called "white coat syndrome". People who have this syndrome may have normal readings when they take their blood pressure on their own.

Three or four out of every ten people with high blood pressure have white coat syndrome, so if you think that you are getting a high blood pressure reading only at the doctor's office, check your blood pressure at home. The best way to diagnose or rule out hypertension is to use a 24-hour blood pressure monitor, which can be requisitioned by your doctor or cardiologist.

Another reason for an inaccurate blood pressure reading is that your doctor may use a blood pressure reading device with a cuff size that is too small. Heavy people with large arms require special large cuffs. The cuff needs to wrap around your arm so that it covers at least 80% of your arm's circumference. If it is too short, you may get a false reading.

The relationship between CVD and diabetes

The relationship between the two is really simple. The primary complication of diabetes is the formation of plaque in the arteries, which can lead to blocked arteries, affecting the heart, the brain and the kidneys. As you will learn later on, both diabetes and CVD have common dietary culprits.

Explore your options and get informed

Getting informed is really important.

As I mentioned already, for decades people have followed the advice of their doctors to reduce dietary saturated fat, cholesterol and salt consumption. Despite this, more people experience a heart attack each year. From 2006 to 2012 alone, the incidence of new heart attacks in the US has gone from 700,000 a year to 785,000 a year. [9,10]

Most people think that it is natural to develop CVD, diabetes or arthritis as they get older. However, all these conditions are preventable! Not only are they preventable, but often these conditions are even reversible! You don't have to lose your health and wellbeing as you get older.

Contrary to popular belief, in most cases it is fairly simple to get your blood pressure and cholesterol under control. It is even possible to reverse the laying down of plaque in your arteries without invasive procedures, so you don't have to suffer a heart attack or a stroke.

CHAPTER 2

RELYING SOLELY ON MEDICATIONS IS DANGEROUS TO YOUR HEALTH

Getting Informed Is Important

When dietary measures to deal with your blood pressure and cholesterol fail (not your fault, since you have been misled), the only other option is to go on medications.

To say that we are an overmedicated society is an understatement. According to the Canadian Institute for Health Information, over two-thirds of Canadians over sixty-five take at least five different drugs, and three of those are for high blood pressure and high cholesterol. In the US, a staggering amount of thirty-one prescriptions are filled each year by those who are sixty-five and older.[11]

In my experience, pharmacists, who are the best trained on the effects of medications on the body, warn against the use of multiple medications at the same time. They call this practice poly-pharmacy. Your pharmacist can be a great resource to get a second opinion from if you are concerned about potential side effects or different drugs interacting with each other in potentially harmful ways.

Most drugs treat symptoms, not disease

Most drugs don't heal disease because they don't treat the cause of disease. For the most part, they only treat the symptoms. A blood pressure pill or a cholesterol pill doesn't reverse hardening and narrowing of the arteries, but, as you will discover shortly, eating the right food and ensuring you get an adequate supply of certain nutrients certainly can.

Let's look briefly at how the most common heart medications work and some of the potential adverse effects they can cause. Then ask yourself a question: if you truly knew what to do, wouldn't you rather rely on food and simple nutritional supplements to resolve your health problems?

Blood pressure medications

To ensure optimal health, the body has various short-term mechanisms to control blood pressure levels. These include hormones and enzymes that affect the removal of salt and water from the kidneys, hormones that affect nervous system control of blood pressure, and the function of minerals, especially calcium and magnesium. Medications used to lower blood pressure manipulate these short-term controls,

9

which are meant to be just that – short term. These meds do nothing to heal the underlying cause of hypertension, which often is the setting in of plaque and stiffness in the arteries. This is probably the reason why blood pressure medications very often stop working after a while, leading your doctor to add one additional medication at a time as a previous drug stops working on its own.

The most popular classes of blood pressure medications are beta blockers, calcium channel blockers, diuretics, angiotensin converting enzyme inhibitors (ACE) and angiotensin receptor blockers.

A recent review of studies on the relationship between drugs for treating mild hypertension (blood pressure up to 159/99) concluded that drug treatment hasn't been shown to reduce mortality (death) or morbidity (injury) of individuals with mild hypertension.[12]

A large study published in the *Journal of the American Medical Association* (JAMA) in 2012 showed no reduction in mortality from cardiovascular events of people taking beta blocker medications for mild to moderate hypertension (blood pressure of up to 200/120).[13]

The "disclaimer" was that the study was an observational study, not a study designed to determine "cause". Nevertheless, the information is quite telling. The key is to treat the cause, not just the symptoms – and most people who follow my dietary and supplementation directives experience an actual *resolution* to hypertension.

Adverse effects of blood pressure medication

The longer a person is on blood pressure medications, the greater the likelihood of developing side effects.

Beta blockers may cause weight gain, impotence, reduced exercise capacity and poor sleep. Long-term use of beta blockers can cause diabetes[14,] and people who take them don't live longer than those who do not take them.[15]

Calcium channel blockers also don't necessarily protect against heart attacks. They may increase the chance of developing congestive heart failure, and people who take these types of meds don't live longer, either.[16, 17]

Diuretic drugs or "water pills" have a mild effect on blood pressure. However, they also cause the elimination of minerals that are vital for cardiovascular health, such as magnesium, potassium and calcium. Thiazide diuretics, a subclass of diuretic medications, deplete potassium and likely increase the risk of developing diabetes.[18]

ACE inhibitors, while considered some of the safest, still have an 11%-17% rate of adverse effects[19] and can potentially speed up kidney damage in diabetics.

Angiotensin receptor blockers should have still fewer side effects than the ACE inhibitors, but the list of these potential adverse effects include dizziness,

11

headaches, high potassium, rash, diarrhea, indigestion, abnormal liver or kidney function, muscle cramps and pain, insomnia, pharyngitis and nasal congestion.[20] Sometimes they can produce an abnormally slow or fast heartbeat and there is controversy over whether they can increase the chance of a heart attack.[21]

A simple Internet search can help you find out which class your medications belong to. Or you can simply ask your pharmacist.

Cholesterol-lowering drugs

As you will discover later on, cholesterol is an extremely important substance for your health, and it can actually be dangerous to limit your body's cholesterol production artificially, particularly with statin drugs.

Statin drugs is a term assigned to the type of drug commonly prescribed to lower cholesterol. All statin drugs do this by blocking a key enzyme involved in the production of cholesterol. This enzyme is called Co HMG reductase. Because of their effect on this enzyme, statin drugs are also known as Co HMG reductase inhibitors. You may know them by their brand names, such as Lipitor, Crestor, Zocor, etc.

Adverse effects of statin drugs
Dr. Beatrice Golomb, MD, PhD, from the University of Los Angeles in San Diego has studied and published a number of papers on the adverse effects of statin

medications. Her research is available on the website *www.statineffects.com*.

These drugs can potentially cause liver and kidney damage, and this can be life threatening. The most commonly reported adverse effects are muscle and joint pain and weakness. Muscles can literally break down, accompanied by feelings of achiness, weakness or tenderness. Other adverse effects include reduction in memory and concentration, depression and irritability, peripheral neuropathy, fatigue and diminished sexual function.

Muscle and nervous system-related symptoms likely result from the effect of statin drugs on Coenzyme Q10 production (CoQ10). These drugs diminish the body's production of this important molecule, which is responsible for energy generation.

The levels of CoQ10 are highest in organs with high rate of metabolism – the liver, brain and...the heart. Therefore, people with low CoQ10 levels are more likely to develop congestive heart failure than people who aren't deficient.

A scientific review published in the medical journal *The Lancet* also revealed an increased incidence of diabetes and hyperglycemia in some people taking these types of drugs.[22] And the FDA (the US Food and Drug Administration) has recently mandated that warnings about the use of statin drugs and risks of developing diabetes and Alzheimer's (memory loss) be placed on the label.

Statin drugs have also been shown to cause cancer in animal models.[23,24]

Why are we (in Western society) over-medicated?

Drug companies are businesses first and foremost. Their mandate isn't to keep people healthy, nor is it to cure people. The mandate of a business is to generate profits.

Unfortunately, the influence drug companies have on doctors and on governments (whose mandate *is* to help people be healthy) is enormous. Because of this influence, the system that is supposed to help us is making us sicker.

Now, don't get me wrong. Most health professionals and people who work in the system are well meaning and do the best they can to help. The conventional medical system works really well for emergency and acute medical care. Unfortunately, it hasn't been as successful at dealing with chronic preventable conditions that are caused by poor dietary and lifestyle choices.

Since most doctors don't offer viable alternatives to the drugs they prescribe, you need to take charge. Get informed and seek out a second opinion. Seek out a medical doctor who is trained in natural medicine, or a licensed naturopathic doctor.

Normalizing blood pressure through the *Healthy Heart Program*

This book will teach you which foods you truly need to avoid and which nutrients you should consume in order to normalize blood pressure and reverse arterial plaque. If you are currently on blood pressure medications, please don't get off these medications all at once without consulting your doctor or naturopathic doctor (regulated as primary healthcare practitioners in many states and provinces).

My experience with my personal patients and the students of *Dr. Klein's Healthy Heart Program*™ is that once they make the nutritional changes required to heal the conditions within their body and within their arteries, they are able to reduce and even eliminate the number and dose of meds they are on. In most cases, the body starts turning itself around very quickly, within weeks – and sometimes within days.

CHAPTER 3

CHOLESTEROL IS YOUR FRIEND, NOT YOUR ENEMY

Cholesterol Does NOT Cause Plaque in the Arteries

The first misconception about cholesterol

The first misconception that I would like to dispel and examine in detail is the idea that cholesterol causes plaque in the arteries. The fact is, cholesterol does NOT cause plaque in the arteries.

This may sound shocking to many readers since for decades now, doctors have attempted to deal with CVD by lowering cholesterol. In fact, cholesterol-lowering medications are some of the most commonly-used types of drugs. Yet the incidence of death from CVD (primarily from heart attacks and strokes) has been relatively unchanged in North America and is growing in the rest of the world.

Not all doctors accept the notion that cholesterol causes cardiovascular disease and leads to blocked arteries. While most medical doctors and the medical system by and large believe that research supports the notion that high cholesterol causes blocked arteries, many other doctors, scientists and researchers don't. Both sides of this debate cite studies to support their arguments.

In a 2009 study, thousands of heart attack patients had their cholesterol levels recorded at the time of the heart attack and 75% of them had normal or low levels of cholesterol![25] If cholesterol truly caused heart attacks, if cholesterol truly clogged up the arteries, wouldn't everyone who suffers a heart attack have a high cholesterol level?

Not only is high cholesterol not the issue, but low cholesterol levels can put you at risk! Sounds outrageous, doesn't it? Well, another study showed that heart attack patients with low levels of cholesterol were twice as likely to die within three years after their cardiac event.[26]

In the ENHANCE trial, the carotid artery thickness (plaque size) was studied in two groups using an ultrasound (an easy, non-invasive procedure). One group received the statin drug Zocor (simvastatin) and the other received Zocor along with Zetia (ezetimibe), a cholesterol absorption blocker. While both medications reduced cholesterol levels, as expected, the combination therapy reduced cholesterol levels the most. Shockingly, subjects in both groups experienced an increase in carotid artery thickness (plaque), with the group that took the combination therapy experiencing the greatest increase in thickness. Again, lowering cholesterol did nothing to reduce the risk for CVD: it actually increased the risk. Surprisingly, even though the combination therapy increased plaque size, the drug was approved for sale and is widely available.[27]

Mature adults are particularly vulnerable to low cholesterol levels. In one study, "each 1 mmol/l increase in total cholesterol corresponded to a 15% decrease in mortality"![28]

In a research paper published by Dr. Elaine M. Meilahn she states:

> "In 1990, an NIH conference concluded from a meta-analysis of 19 studies that men and, to a lesser extent, women with a total serum cholesterol level below 4.2 mmol/l (160 mg/dl) (6th percentile) exhibited about a 10% to 20% *excess* total mortality compared with those with a cholesterol level between 4.2 and 5.2 mmol/l (160 to 199 mg/dl). Specifically, excess causes of death included cancer (primarily lung and hematopoietic), respiratory and digestive disease, violent death (suicide and trauma), and hemorrhagic stroke."
> [29]

18

In a more recent study, individuals between the ages of sixty and eight-five (average age was seventy-one) were followed for twelve years. Those individuals with cholesterol levels of more than 200 mg/dl or 5.2 mmol/l showed a 24% reduced risk of mortality over the study period. Lower cholesterol levels (less than 170 mg/dl or 4.4 mmol/l) were associated with a 60% increased risk of death![30]

A study used by the medical establishment to promote their claim that cholesterol causes heart attacks is the Framingham Heart Study. This observational study, the longest one of its kind, started in the late forties and is still going today. It is named after the town of Framingham, Massachusetts, where researchers have been following many of its residents in order to discover which factors contribute to CVD and which factors protect against CVD.

Although the study did find an association between high levels of blood cholesterol and increased likelihood of future heart attacks, the elevated cholesterol was only one of over 240 "risk factors" that were associated with increased risk of heart attack. And in fact, this association was found *only* in young and middle-aged men, not older men, nor in women of any age group. In the thirty-year follow-up of the Framingham study, high cholesterol was not predictive of heart attack at all after the age of forty-seven. In other words, according to the Framingham study, once a man reached the age of forty-eight there was *no* relationship between high levels of cholesterol and dying of a heart attack.

More alarming was the fact that those whose cholesterol dropped without any intervention ran a much higher risk of heart attack than those whose cholesterol increased. The significantly-increased risk of dying from CVD and from other diseases in those whose cholesterol decreased was contrary to what we have been led to believe. This information came from an article that appeared in the prestigious *Journal of the American Medical Association* on April 24, 1987 under the title "Cholesterol and mortality. Thirty years of follow-up from the Framingham study". Its authors were the chief investigators of the Framingham study at the time, W.P. Castelli, K.M. Anderson, and D. Levy.[31]

There are many published studies, discussion papers and books about this topic. You can find some of them on my website *www.drkleinhealthyheart.com.*

Cholesterol is necessary for optimal health

Cholesterol is a lipid, a fatty substance that is absolutely necessary for optimal health. About 85% of your cholesterol is made by your body because it needs it! Why would the human body produce so much cholesterol if it was bad for us?

Some of the common reasons that your body makes and needs cholesterol are discussed below.

Cholesterol is present in all cell membranes.

Our body is made of hundreds of trillions of cells. Each cell is like an office building or a factory, buzzing with the metabolic activities needed to keep us alive and healthy. The cell membrane is like the wall of these "buildings". Cell membranes must be strong yet flexible. They need to protect the cell from harmful outside influences, while allowing necessary substances through. Cholesterol plays a crucial role in maintaining the strength and flexibility of cell membranes. Without it, cell membranes become too rigid and are unable to carry out their function properly. As a result, cells break down and die.

Cholesterol is a precursor of steroid hormones.

Cholesterol is the raw material the body uses to make steroid hormones.

- *Estrogen* is a sex hormone produced in the ovaries and adrenal gland. It is mostly known for its responsibility for the development of the female sex organs. Estrogen is also important for maintaining healthy skin and blood vessels, strong bones, a balance in blood fluidity, proper hydration (water) in the body, and high HDL ("good cholesterol"). Having too little estrogen can affect all of these health factors, while having too much can increase the "stickiness of blood" and increase blood lipids such as triglycerides. Estrogen levels diminish substantially after menopause, thus increasing the risk for CVD.

Adequate cholesterol levels while aging are important to help the body maximize its production of estrogen.

- *Progesterone* is involved in regulating the menstrual cycle and pregnancy. Progesterone also has multiple effects outside of the reproductive system. It relaxes the muscles and lungs and regulates mucus. It acts as an anti-inflammatory agent and assists in maintaining a healthy immune system. Progesterone also normalizes blood clotting and vascular tone, zinc and copper levels, cell oxygen levels, and use of fat stores for energy. In addition, progesterone assists in thyroid function, in bone building and in regulating nerve function. Progesterone appears to prevent endometrial cancer and other reproductive organs cancers (involving the uterus) by countering the effect of too much estrogen.

- *Testosterone* is another sex hormone, mostly known for its role in the development of male sex organs and male vitality. In male adults, it is important for maintaining strong muscle mass and bones, healthy sex drive and libido, and mental (mood) and physical strength (good energy levels). Clearly, when cholesterol levels are too low all of these health factors suffer.

- *Cortisol* is a very important hormone for stress adaptation and for regulating inflammation. It suppresses immune response in case of too much inflammation or allergies. It also regulates blood pressure, in part by controlling sodium balance.

- *Aldosterone* is a hormone that acts on the kidneys to retain salt, water and proper electrolyte balance in the body and to help regulate blood pressure. It also helps regulate the acid/alkaline balance in the body.

- *Vitamin D* is a hormone/vitamin with vast health benefits. It plays a role in the health of bones, the immune system and the cardiovascular system, as well as cancer prevention.

Cholesterol is needed for making bile and bile acids

Bile and bile acids assist in digesting fats, oils and fat-soluble vitamins (vitamins, A, D, E and K). It is also needed for the production of vitamin D in the body, and vitamin D is important for ensuring healthy bones, immune system, nervous system, and much more.

As you can see from all the important roles that cholesterol plays, simply slashing its levels in the blood through medications can have a harmful impact on your health.

"Bad" cholesterol versus "good cholesterol", and other lipids

Low Density Lipoprotein (LDL, or "bad cholesterol") and High Density Lipoprotein (HDL, or "good cholesterol") are not different types of cholesterol. These terms simply refer to the types of transport vehicles involved in carrying cholesterol away from the cells through the blood vessels and then back into cells.

Cholesterol is a lipid, an oil. Water and oil don't mix. So in order for cholesterol, which is oily, to travel in the blood, which is mostly water, it needs to be carried by something else that is soluble in water. The body has created special water-soluble proteins to transport cholesterol in the blood stream. These are called transport proteins. When such a protein is attached to cholesterol or to other lipids, the entire structure is called a lipoprotein.

The following types of lipids commonly appear on your blood test report and the test for these lipids is called a "lipid panel".

Low Density Lipoprotein (LDL) is the major carrier of cholesterol away from the liver and other cells, where it is made, through the blood to other areas in the body, where it is needed. LDL is considered "bad" due to the false belief that having a lot of it circulating in the blood can cause plaque. However, as mentioned earlier, most heart attack patients have normal cholesterol levels. If LDL truly caused plaque, then every person who succumbs to a heart attack or a stroke would have high LDL cholesterol.

According to conventional medicine, LDL cholesterol levels are considered high when levels excess 129mg/dl or 3.3mmol/l for most people. (Mmol measures apply to Canada & most of Europe.)

High Density Lipoprotein (HDL): This carrier takes cholesterol away from various parts of the body and the blood vessels back into the liver and other cells, where it can be reutilized or excreted (leave the body) in bile into the intestines and out during a bowel movement. It also carries antioxidant enzymes and vitamins that prevent the oxidation of cholesterol. This is why it is important that HDL levels remain healthy. You will soon learn about the role of oxidation in cardiovascular disease.

HDL cholesterol is considered normal at levels higher than 40-49mg/dl (1-1.3 mmol/l) for men and 50-59mg/dl (1.3-1.5mmol/l) for women. However, more desirable are levels greater than 60mg/dl (1.6mmol/l).

Very Low Density Lipoprotein (VLDL): Like LDL, VLDL is a carrier of cholesterol and fats in the blood stream. VLDL is generally converted into LDL. It can get oxidized easily, which can be a problem, as you will learn soon.

Total cholesterol is the combination of LDL, HDL and VLDL.

In conventional medicine, cholesterol levels are considered too high when total cholesterol levels are greater than 200mg/dl (5.2mmol/l).

Triglycerides are not cholesterol. However, whenever your doctor tests your cholesterol, he or she also tests your triglycerides. A triglyceride is basically three molecules of fat attached together to the backbone of a molecule called glycerol. This is how your body "packages" fat. High amounts of triglycerides in the arteries are related to an increased risk of heart attack and stroke. Healthy triglyceride levels are below 150mg/dl (1.7mmol/l).

Total Cholesterol to HDL ratio: This ratio, calculated by dividing total cholesterol by HDL, is a better indicator of CVD risk than total cholesterol and the ideal ratio sought after is between 3.5:1 and 5:1.

Regardless of all this info, it is important not to get hung up on cholesterol as a risk factor.

Getting the right perspective

Since I started my practice, I have often spoken to patients who themselves, or someone close to them, experienced a heart attack or a stroke despite having a "normal" cholesterol level.

I have also treated individuals who had familial hypercholesterolemia, a relatively infrequent genetic condition of very high cholesterol levels, who had completely clean arteries and were very healthy.

The most important substances on the lipid panel that are predictive of CVD are HDL, triglycerides and the total cholesterol to HDL ratio. You want to make sure your triglycerides are low enough and that your HDL is sufficiently high. This book will discuss these and other predictive factors of cardiovascular disease later on.

Now, cholesterol does not just stick to arteries to form plaque. To understand this, it is helpful to consider the physical properties of cholesterol. If cholesterol was the cause of plaque in the arteries, it would have to be a sticky substance, able to stick to the arterial wall. However, cholesterol is an oil and oils are not sticky, oils are slippery. In fact, cholesterol is used by cosmetic product manufacturers as a foundation for creams and to assist in the absorption of creams and other cosmetic preparations. So cholesterol on its own doesn't just stick to the arteries.

A sticky kind of cholesterol

Recently, scientists did discover a sticky kind of low density lipoprotein (LDL). It is called MGmin low density lipoprotein.[32]

Do you know what makes it sticky? Sugar. Sugar is a sticky, glue-like substance. Blood levels of MGmin cholesterol are particularly high in diabetics, who have high levels of sugar circulating in their arteries. MGmin cholesterol is not present in high amounts in the blood stream of non-diabetics. Of course, CVD is the primary complication of diabetes.

This type of cholesterol *is* associated with atherosclerosis and plaque. However, it is the presence of *sugar* in the blood (from food), and the sticking of sugar to LDL cholesterol, that produces MGmin LDL. People with low cholesterol levels who consume lots of sugar are still likely to have too much MGmin LDL and are at a higher risk.

Since cholesterol is so vital to your health and since it doesn't cause cardiovascular disease, it is senseless to worry about high cholesterol levels. Instead, you need to make sure your cholesterol levels don't drop too low and, more important, as you will read in a few chapters, you need to watch your blood sugar levels and sugar intake.

CHAPTER 4

SATURATED FAT – A BIG FAT LIE

Saturated fat is NOT dangerous, contrary to what you have been lead to believe!

The purpose of this chapter is to provide evidence to dispel the commonly-held and wrongly popularized misconception that the consumption of saturated fat causes CVD.

Before I start discussing the scientific evidence that supports this idea and the health benefits of saturated fats, it would be useful to have a basic understanding of what fats and oils are and what the difference is between saturated and unsaturated oils. This will also allow you to understand later on what makes these two different types of oil healthy or harmful.

The basic structure of fats / oils

Fats and oils are almost one and the same in terms of their chemical structure and biological function. They both belong to a class of substances called lipids. The difference between fats and oils is whether they are solid or liquid at room temperature. Fats tend to be solid at room temperature, while oils are liquid at room temperature.

The basic structure of fats and oils consists of a chain or a "skeleton" of carbon atoms, to which hydrogen atoms are bound. Every carbon in a fat molecule has the potential to bind two hydrogen atoms. If every carbon in the "chain" is indeed bound to two hydrogen atoms, the structure is said to be "saturated". It is saturated by hydrogen atoms and no other hydrogen atoms or atoms of any kind have any room to join the fat molecule. This saturation with hydrogen atoms makes it solid at room temperature.

On the other hand, when hydrogen atoms are missing from a single pair of two adjacent carbon atoms on the chain, the lipid is said to be "monounsaturated" ("mono" refers to the single pair of carbon atoms). When hydrogen atoms are missing from multiple pairs of adjacent carbon atoms, the lipid is polyunsaturated ("poly" refers to more than one pair of carbon atoms). Monounsaturated and poly unsaturated oils tend to exist as a liquid at room temperature.

The image on the next page is a visual tool to help you understand the difference between saturated fat and mono and poly unsaturated oil.

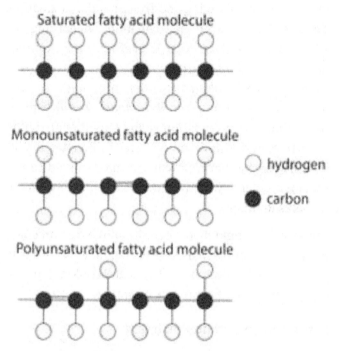

Animals and plants generally contain all three types of oils, saturated, monounsaturated and polyunsaturated. Plants contain mostly mono and poly unsaturated oil. Animals, however, have significantly more saturated fat than plants do. The exception is coconuts and palm kernels, with over ninety percent saturated fat content. Common sources of dietary saturated fat include butter, cream, eggs, tallow and suet (beef fat), lard, as well as coconuts and palm kernel oil.

READ THIS IF YOU HAVE A HEART

The more unsaturated oil is (the more hydrogen atoms it "lacks") the more structurally unstable and more harmful it is. It can be easily destroyed by excessive heat (cooking and frying) and by oxidation. This is called lipid peroxidation. According to Wikipedia, "*Lipid peroxidation refers to the oxidative degradation of lipids. It is the process in which free radicals "steal" electrons from the lipids in cell membranes, resulting in cell damage*". I will explain more about what oxidation is and how it contributes to CVD, hypertension and diabetes in Chapter 6, and will discuss the harm polyunsaturated oils do to the cardiovascular system and their contribution to diabetes in Chapter 7.

The complete binding or saturation of a carbon chain by hydrogen atoms makes saturated fat very stable. It can't be easily destroyed by heat (cooking) or by oxidation and so it cannot be harmful.

Saturated fat and human health

We need saturated fat for good health. Just as the human body contains significant amounts of cholesterol, it also naturally contains even a greater amount of saturated fat. Out of the three types of fat in the human body, the greatest amount (about 45%) is saturated and the balance consists of monounsaturated and polyunsaturated fatty acids.

The following information about the importance of saturated fat to human health is an excerpt from an article called "The Skinny on Fat",[33] written by Dr. Mary Enig, PhD of the Weston A. Price Foundation.

- "Saturated fatty acids constitute at least 50% of the cell membranes. They give our cells necessary stiffness and integrity.

- They play a vital role in the health of our bones. For calcium to be effectively incorporated into the skeletal structure, at least 50% of the dietary fats should be saturated.

- They lower Lp(a), a substance in the blood that indicates proneness to heart disease.

- They protect the liver from alcohol and other toxins, such as Tylenol.

- They enhance the immune system.

- They are needed for the proper utilization of essential fatty acids. Elongated omega 3 fatty acids are better retained in the tissues when the diet is rich in saturated fats.

- Saturated 18-carbon stearic acid and 16-carbon palmitic acid are the preferred foods for the heart, which is why the fat around the heart

READ THIS IF YOU HAVE A HEART

muscle is highly saturated. The
heart draws on this reserve of fat in
times of stress.

- Short- and medium-chain saturated
  fatty acids have important
  antimicrobial properties. They
  protect us against harmful
  microorganisms in the digestive
  tract."

Evidence that saturated fat doesn't cause CVD

An important consideration is that while the
consumption of saturated fat has decreased
significantly over the last hundred years, the
incidence of CVD has significantly increased. The
graph on the following page [34] shows how the
consumption of saturated fat in the US went down
from between 12.5 pounds and 15 pounds per year in
the early part of the twentieth century to well below
5 pounds by the end of the twentieth century. Early
in the twentieth century most people lived on a farm
and they cooked with butter, cream, beef, pork and
poultry fat. Over the past one hundred years, the use
of polyunsaturated seed oils has gone up
significantly. Common sources of polyunsaturated
oils include cotton seeds, canola (rape seeds), soy
beans, safflower seeds, sunflower seeds, etc.

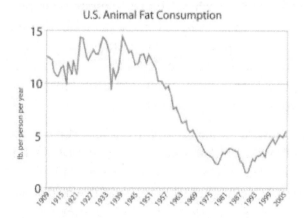

Throughout the same period of time the incidence of CVD increased from less than 9% in 1909 to upwards of 30% when it reached its peak in the nineteen fifties and sixties.[35] So how can it possibly be that saturated fat causes CVD?

This trend continues into the early part of the 21st century. Data tracking fat consumption from the 1960s to the late 1990s shows a significant reduction in saturated fat consumption accompanied by a continuous increase in the incidence of heart attacks and obesity. [36, 37, 38]

Where do doctors who advise us to avoid saturated fat get their information from? You'd expect that their view would be based on sound research, the kind of high-quality research that gets published in well-known scientific and medical journals.

Well, guess what most research about this topic reveals? In the last several years alone, three scientific reviews showed that saturated fat does NOT cause CVD.[39,40,41] As I mentioned in the last chapter, a scientific review is a study that analyzes data from numerous studies. So the three reviews I reference here altogether account for tens, if not hundreds of studies about this topic.

The following is an excerpt from an article called "The Truth about Saturated Fat" by Mary Enig, PhD and Sally Fallon (Weston A. Price Foundation). The authors give examples from around the world of how various levels of saturated fat consumptions in different culture influence their health.

> "Numerous surveys of traditional populations have yielded information that is an embarrassment to the Diet Dictocrats. For example, a study comparing Jews when they lived in Yemen, whose diets contained fats solely of animal origin, to Yemenite Jews living in Israel, whose diets contained margarine and vegetable oils, revealed little heart disease or diabetes in the former group but high levels of both diseases in the latter. (The study also noted that the Yemenite Jews consumed no sugar but those in Israel consumed sugar in amounts equaling 25-30% of total carbohydrate intake.)

A comparison of populations in northern and southern India revealed a similar pattern. People in northern India consume 17 times more animal fat but have an incidence of coronary heart disease seven times lower than people in southern India. The Masai and kindred tribes of Africa subsist largely on milk, blood and beef. They are free from coronary heart disease and have excellent blood cholesterol levels.

Eskimos eat liberally of animal fats from fish and marine animals. On their native diet they are free of disease and exceptionally hardy. An extensive study of diet and disease patterns in China found that the region in which the populace consumes large amounts of whole milk had half the rate of heart disease as several districts in which only small amounts of animal products are consumed.

Several Mediterranean societies have low rates of heart disease even though fat – including highly saturated fat from lamb, sausage and goat cheese – comprises up to 70% of their caloric intake. The inhabitants of Crete, for example, are remarkable for their good health and longevity. A study of Puerto Ricans revealed that, although they consume large amounts of animal fat, they have a very low incidence of colon and breast cancer.

A study of the long-lived inhabitants of Soviet Georgia revealed that those who eat the most fatty meat live the longest. In Okinawa, where the average life span for women is 84 years – longer than in Japan – the inhabitants eat generous amounts of pork and seafood and do all their cooking in lard. None of these studies is mentioned by those urging restriction of saturated fats." [42]

As you can see, the scientific evidence about the safety, health benefits and importance of saturated fat is overwhelming. We need to embrace butter, cream, eggs, animal fat and coconut oil as health foods. Saturated fat is important for human health and eating less and less of it has cost us our health. Animal fat does not cause cardiovascular disease.[43] Generally, dietary sources of saturated fat are also good sources of some important fat soluble vitamins (vitamins that exist in fat), particularly vitamins A, D and K, all of which contribute to good health, including optimal cardiovascular health.

However, it is important to mention that the only sources of saturated fat that are linked to CVD are processed meats such as luncheon meats, cold cuts, sausages and other types of meats prepared with additives and preservatives.

Now let's explore another misconception.

CHAPTER 5

TOO LITTLE SALT CAN BE DANGEROUS TO YOUR HEALTH

Salt is Necessary to Human Health

The "war" against salt

The "war" against salt, or more specifically sodium, has been another folly. The body needs salt (both sodium and chloride). Public health agencies have been pushing a low salt agenda, claiming that restricting sodium intake to less than 2300mg a day (less than a teaspoon) will save lives by reducing hypertension and CVD. This is based on an understanding of salt physiology that explains that too much salt in the circulation leads to an increase in the volume of water in the blood vessels (salt attracts water). An increase in water volume and blood volume would raise blood pressure. However, what is not considered is that sodium doesn't simply accumulate in the blood vessels because excessive salt is removed by the kidneys (except in people with chronic renal failure).

For decades, mountains of research have refuted the assumption that limiting salt decreases blood pressure and prevents CVD. Most studies point out that the 1.5 to 2 teaspoons most populations in the world consume seem to serve them well. One teaspoon holds 6.2g (6200mg) of salt. If you consider that table salt consists of 40% sodium and 60% chloride, 2300mg of sodium amount to less than a teaspoon of salt, which is less than what most people in the world eat.

Here are some key areas of your health that sodium and chloride are important for.

Sodium is important for:

- Regulation of blood pressure and flexibility of the arteries

- A healthy nervous system; sodium is required for nerve conduction

- Helping with the passage of various nutrients such as carbohydrates, calcium and vitamin C, into the cells

- The production of various hormones needed to sustain and maintain life, particularly a number of hormones produced in the adrenal gland

Chloride is important for:

- Maintaining healthy blood volume and blood pressure

- Helping to regulate a healthy acid/alkaline balance in the body (a slight deviation can be fatal)

- Healthy muscle activity

- Movement of water into and out of cells, which is extremely important for hydration

- Needed for producing hydrochloric acid necessary for optimal digestion of food, especially protein.

Not only is salt important for your health, I would argue that consuming more than 2300mg of sodium will likely do nothing to your blood pressure; in fact, limiting it can sometimes raise your blood pressure. Read the following examples and decide for yourself.

Salt and blood pressure

In the Intersalt study [44], conducted in the late 1980s, the impact of salt on the health of fifty-six different populations around the world was examined. These populations consumed between 1.5 to 2 teaspoons of salt per day. In fifty-two of these populations salt consumption did nothing to blood pressure either way. In fact, those who ate the most salt had a LOWER median blood pressure than those who ate the least salt. Unfortunately, the researchers based their conclusions on only four populations out of the fifty-six studied. In these four, significantly low consumption of salt was associated with significantly lower blood pressure.[45]

Another study showed that significantly limiting salt consumption produced a slight reduction in blood pressure in 30% of the study's subjects, but increased it in 20% of the subjects and did nothing to the remaining 50%.[46]

A 1991 study showed that 7.2 g of salt is the minimum amount of salt people need. Researchers found that intakes of less than 120 mmol (2760mg) per day of sodium, the amount found in 7.2g of salt, caused plasma rennin levels to spike and signaled the rennin-angiotensin-aldosterone system (RAS) to recoup sodium from the kidneys. Increase in the hormones renin, angiotensin and aldosterone is closely associated with increase in blood pressure. [47] An increase in these hormones promotes insulin resistance, which leads to poor blood sugar regulation, a factor that is closely related to atherosclerosis and CVD

Another thing to consider is that while salt consumption has remained flat for the past forty years, the incidence of hypertension has continued to increase during that period of time.

Focusing on salt reduction takes the focus away from more important factors. Not only does its reduction have a weak relationship with blood pressure reduction, limiting salt can have an adverse effect on the prevention of cardiovascular disease and longevity.

Salt, your cardiovascular wellbeing and your overall health

The following studies show the importance of salt to our health and the danger of restricting it.

Data from the National Health and Nutrition Examination Surveys[48,49, 50] shows that low salt diets are associated with a slight *increase* in mortality from all causes. In other words, people on a low salt diet don't live as long as people who don't follow a low salt diet.

An analysis of 167 studies showed that salt reduction increased risk factors associated with CVD.[51]

A 2008 study showed that salt restriction increased levels of inflammation in the body, another factor that is closely related to atherosclerosis and CVD.[52]

These are just a few examples of research that refutes the idea that current salt consumption is dangerous to human health. If anything, salt restriction is dangerous to human health.

What needs to be considered is the source of our salt. Some of the most common dietary sources of salt include bread, pizza, processed meats, chips, etc. Later you will see that these foods' have potential for harm for reasons other than the salt they contain.

Now let's get down to the real culprits of CVD.

CHAPTER 6

REFINED CARBS – A FATAL ATTRACTION

One of the Two Worst Culprits of CVD

A 2009 scientific review of many studies on the relationship between diet and cardiovascular disease concluded that foods with a high glycemic index or glycemic load were one of the two worst culprits of CVD.[53] (The second culprit is discussed in the next chapter).

Glycemic index refers to how quickly blood sugar levels (i.e. levels of glucose in the blood) rise after eating a particular type of food. Glycemic load estimates how much the food will raise a person's blood glucose level after eating it. One unit of glycemic load approximates the effect of consuming one gram of glucose.

Most us are careful not to eat butter and meat (which, as you learned, don't cause cardiovascular disease), yet we eat far more sugar than people have ever eaten. The average North American eats about twenty-two or more teaspoons of sugar daily.

Commercially-made foods all have lots of sugar added. We also get lots of sugar from starchy food, especially baked goods. When digested, starch turns into sugar, specifically glucose. So when we eat a typical North American diet we get huge amounts of sugar. We get it from any of the following types of food: breakfast cereals, bread (even whole wheat or multi grain), bagels, pizza, any baked goods, jam, honey, any processed spreads, candies and candy bars, ice cream, juices and sodas, rice, potatoes, corn, "low fat" yogurts and many processed foods.

The two most common types of sugar we consume are glucose and fructose. Both of them, in the right amount and with the availability of certain vitamins and minerals, are metabolized to produce the energy we need to live. However, when we consume too much glucose and fructose from foods that don't contain adequate amounts of vitamins and minerals, these foods, as you will shortly see, can become harmful.

The dangers of high fructose corn syrup (HFCS)

Fructose in fruit is generally healthy. However, most of the fructose Westerners eat comes from either refined sucrose (table sugar) or from high-fructose corn syrup (HFCS). Both are devoid of important vitamins and minerals. Without these vitamins and minerals the body is unable to use these types of sugar productively, to turn the sugar into energy.

While both table sugar and HFCS have an equal amount of glucose and fructose, HFCS is twenty times sweeter, is cheaper to make and is addictive. Worse, it contains 5 times the amount of carbohydrates than what is actually listed on the label.[54]

Why this discrepancy? HFCS comes from cornstarch, and much of that starch is unaccounted for on the labels of the foods and beverages that contain HFCS. So, when you drink a carbonated drink containing HFCS, you may be getting five times the amount of sugar listed on the label!

HFCS also contains a substance called carbonyl, a free radical that causes tissue damage.

Because HFCS is cheaper and sweeter than sucrose, the food industry uses more HFCS than table sugar, and you can find it in many, many foods and beverages.

While glucose can be metabolized and turned into energy in various organs in the body, fructose is metabolized mainly in the liver. Too much fructose and glucose are turned into fat (triglycerides and VLDL – very low density lipoprotein) and cause insulin resistance, as well as a condition called fatty liver (lots of fat in liver cells), which is closely related to CVD. As you will soon read, both these types of sugar "caramelize" the arteries.

Insulin resistance

Glucose requires insulin in order to get absorbed by the cells. Therefore, too much sugar (without an adequate supply of vitamins and minerals) can result in too much insulin production. This, in turn, can lead to a number of health issues, including diabetes, inflammation, cancer and poor metabolism.

In one "accidental" experiment in the early seventies by Dr. Cruz, the dripping of insulin on a dog's artery in a lab caused an almost complete occlusion (blockage) within three months.

"Insulin resistance" is a condition caused by consuming excessive amounts of both types of sugar, glucose and fructose. Other causes of insulin resistance include overeating, consuming too much polyunsaturated oil and having an inadequate supply of certain vitamins and minerals needed to facilitate cellular absorption and utilization of nutrients, especially sugar.

It is a condition in which, after years of over exposure to insulin, our cells become resistant to the effect of insulin. If insulin can't do its job, glucose can't enter the cells efficiently to be used up for energy production, so some of it lingers in the blood vessels, causing harm and leading to plaque build-up.

How sugar causes plaque in the arteries

Most people who eat a modern Western type of diet get too much sugar in the arteries. Sugar causes plaque in the arteries in two main ways: through glycation and oxidation.

Glycation (stickiness)

You've probably noticed that when you touch candy, honey or anything rich in sugar, the sugar you touch sticks to your hands and stays there until you wash it off. Sugar, by nature, is sticky, and when too much of it lingers in your arteries, it simply sticks to the arteries. Although clogging of the arteries is the most common complication of diabetes, you don't need to be diabetic for your arteries to accumulate plaque. Hypothyroidism, stress, deficiencies of various vitamins and minerals and other common factors can diminish or slow down the transport of sugar into the cells, keeping more of it in the arteries, where it can stick to the arterial wall.

The scientific term for this process is glycation. Once the arteries become sticky from the glucose that gets attached to them, other "stuff"– various types of proteins, fats, minerals and other molecules – can stick to them. The scientific term assigned to the binding of sugar to other "stuff" is called advanced glycation end products (AGE products). This is the beginning of plaque.

Through the process of sugar binding or sticking to different substances, not only do you get the beginning of plaque formation, other processes occur that make things worse. Certain immune molecules can bind to the sugar on the arteries. This contributes to inflammation, which makes the plaque grow and makes the blood "thick". [55, 56, 57]

Sugar can also bind a tiny molecule called nitric oxide, which is in charge of keeping the arteries relaxed and dilated. When levels of nitric oxide decline, the arteries constrict and become narrowed. This decreases blood flow in the arteries and can contribute to high blood pressure.

It is surprising how little we hear about the dangers of glycation as a causative factor in CVD, because considering and addressing glycation as a cause of CVD is so much more relevant than cholesterol.

Oxidation

The presence of excessive sugar also brings about hardening of the arteries by causing oxidation. Sugar isn't the only culprit; other foods and substances, such as polyunsaturated oil and its derivatives hydrogenated oil and trans fats, as well as cigarette smoke, can also cause oxidation.

In chemical terms, oxidation refers to the transfer of electrons or oxygen from one substance or molecule to another. This happens all the time in our cells as a part of the different metabolic (life) processes. However, excessive oxidation damages cells and structures in the body. It damages structures such as cell membranes, protein and DNA, causing degeneration and cellular aging. It can also rob our cells of vital energy. The arteries are made of cells and rope like protein fibers. Excessive oxidation leads to stiffening of the arteries, and as flexibility is lost, blood pressure rises. Oxidation also contributes to plaque development and to narrowing of the arteries, which affects circulation.

A common example of oxidation you may be familiar with is the rusting of metal that is caused by its exposure to oxygen in air or in water. Imagine a thin and flexible metal wire which becomes rusted over the years. Once rust is extensive, it becomes rigid and loses its flexibility and if you bend it, it would snap because rust weakens the structure.

Both glycation and oxidation damage the arteries and are the main ways atherosclerosis happens. Any time damage occurs, the body strives to repair the damage through a process called inflammation. Inflammation is a double-edged sword. Short-term inflammation which is able to lead to complete repair of the arteries can help us heal and prevent CVD, while long-term, on-going inflammation, without proper repair, is deadly.

More on inflammation later. First, let's find out what the next most harmful dietary substance is.

CHAPTER 7

AVOID THESE OILS

The Second Culprit of CVD

Polyunsaturated fatty acid oils (PUFA)

The other major dietary cause of CVD is polyunsaturated fatty acids that people consume mostly from seed oils such as canola oil (rape seed oil), corn oil, cotton seed oil, sunflower seed oil, safflower oil, soy oil and grape seed oil. Recall that in Chapter Four I explained that polyunsaturated fatty acid is an oil that is missing hydrogen atoms at more than one location on the oil molecule; as a result, it is unstable and prone to destruction from oxidation and heat. There are two major sub classifications of polyunsaturated fatty acid oils (PUFA). The first is called omega three polyunsaturated fatty acid (also known as omega three essential fatty acid). The other is called omega six polyunsaturated fatty acid (also known as omega six essential fatty acid). The seed oils are generally a source of the omega six oils, while animal fat, especially fish and sea animals, are a source of omega three oils.

For decades the public has been misled to believe that the PUFA seed oils are protective against heart disease and that they promote health. This idea served the commercial food industry and the seed oil companies, who, in the early part of the twentieth century started replacing the traditional animal fats used to cook and fry food with the cheaper-to-manufacture seed oils. Studies that were funded by huge seed oil companies[58] and studies that were poorly done[59] showed that seed oil based omega six oils were the best thing you could consume for your heart. These studies often claimed to compare the impact on health of saturated fat versus PUFA. Yet the saturated fat sources that many of these studies analyzed often included the undisclosed presence of the highly unhealthy trans fats. When you lump saturated fat and harmful trans fat into a single category labeled "saturated fat", it is easy to produce harmful effects on cardiovascular health.[60] On the other hand, other well designed, impartial studies, including large scientific reviews, showed that replacing the combined group of saturated fat and trans fats with omega six PUFA increased the risk of CVD by 13%! Note that even when the harmful trans fats were lumped together with saturated fat, omega six PUFA still fared worse.

This increased risk for CVD was reduced by 22% when the omega six PUFA oils were combined with omega three PUFA oils.[61]

It is interesting that when in one study the oil / fat content of arterial plaque was examined, most of it consisted of omega six PUFA, which comes predominately from those so called "healthy" seed based "vegetable" oils. Incidentally, only 26% of the fat in the plaque was in the form of saturated fat.[62]

When PUFA provide more than 4% of our caloric daily intake (simply put, when consumed excessively as they have been for many decades now in the West), they promote inflammation and the onset of CVD, as well as diabetes, cancer and other diseases.[63, 64, 65, 66]

How PUFA contribute to CVD and disease in general

There are two or three primary ways by which PUFA contribute to the development of CVD and poor health in general.

The first one is oxidation. In Chapter 4 I explained that due to the structural characteristics of polyunsaturated fatty acid, it is an unstable oil that can be easily damaged by heat and oxidation. Once it becomes oxidized, it too can become an oxidizing agent. As an oxidizing agent it contributes to oxidation of the arteries, which stiffens the arteries. The body's response is an attempt to repair and so inflammation sets in, which contributes to plaque development and growth.

PUFA also contribute to the oxidation of cholesterol, which is implicated in plaque development.[67, 68]

What I am going to share with you next is the best explanation I have come across to date to explain the presence of cholesterol in arterial plaque. Remember, I explained earlier that almost every cell in the body makes cholesterol. White blood cells also make cholesterol. This cholesterol leaves the cell when it is needed elsewhere. The function of white blood cells at the site of plaque is to remove any debris and damaged substances by swallowing and degrading these substances. These cells also swallow oxidized cholesterol. Researchers discovered that the oxidized cholesterol white blood cells swallow interferes with the exit of the healthy cholesterol the white blood cells produce on their own. As a result, they keep on accumulating both types of cholesterol until the cells burst and empty their content, all that cholesterol, at the site of the plaque.[69,70]

PUFA also damage the arteries and causes CVD and other diseases through glycation. I described glycation as a process that makes the arteries sticky in the last chapter. Now, you thought sugar was bad? Glycation through lipid (PUFA) oxidation causes glycation of the arteries twenty-three times faster than simple sugars do![71] So the faster the artery becomes sticky the faster plaque develops.

Just like high glycemic carbs, only in a more potent way, PUFA contribute to oxidation and glycation of the arteries, leading to plaque development and possibly to blockages of the arteries.

Hydrogenated oil and trans fatty acid

Even worse than polyunsaturated oil are its derivatives, partially hydrogenated oil and trans fatty acid.

Partially hydrogenated oil and trans fat is made when a polyunsaturated seed oil is placed in a closed chamber where it is flooded by hydrogen gas under a condition of high heat and high pressure. The hydrogen atoms bind to the polyunsaturated seed oil, partially saturating it. The resulting product is a partially saturated oil, also known as partially hydrogenated oil, with a semi- solid consistency like soft butter. Under these conditions, some of the bonds between neighboring carbon atoms in the "spine" of the oil become bent. The resulting different shape of the newly formed oil is referred to by chemists as a "trans" shape, hence the term "trans" fat.

Hydrogenated oil and trans fat are commonly found in margarine, which constitutes a convenient and cheap substitute for butter. It is also widely used in snack food items, fast foods, fried foods and baked food items. Hydrogenated oil has been widely used in these types of foods for two primary reasons. They increase the shelf life of food, often eliminating the need for refrigeration, and they are cheaper than saturated animal fat.

However, hydrogenated oil – and especially trans fat – is extremely harmful to human health. According to a scientific review I quoted earlier, along with high glycemic foods, trans fat is a leading cause of CVD.[72]

According to an article by University of Illinois researcher Fred Kummerow, published in the medical journal *Atherosclerosis*, trans fat contributes to plaque built up and the formation of blood clots in several ways.[73]

Trans fat stimulates an increase of LDL cholesterol and, just like polyunsaturated oil, contributes to the oxidation of LDL cholesterol and the oxidation of the arteries.

Trans fat also interferes with enzymes that control blood flow and blood clotting.

When you shop for food, make sure to read labels to find out if trans fatty acids, hydrogenated oil or partially hydrogenated oil are present. As well, beware of hidden amounts: commercially-made foods with less than half a gram of trans fat per serving aren't required to list it on the label.

Now you know which dietary factors cause CVD and which don't cause CVD. Later, we'll put it together and discuss what a heart-healthy diet should consist of.

CHAPTER 8

INFLAMMATION – YOUR BODY IS TRYING TO HELP YOU

How the Body Attempts to Heal Itself

Inflammation is a process of repair

Any time structures or tissues in the body get damaged, including the arteries, the body attempts to repair the damaged structures. This process of repair is called inflammation. It is the body's attempt to heal itself. Typical signs of inflammation are swelling, redness, heat and sometimes pain. Basically, all of these signs are the result of increased circulation to the site of damage or injury.

If the body is able to carry out the repair to its completion, the inflammation subsides as the tissue or structure is healed (repaired). If the body is unable to carry out the repair to its completion, inflammation persists and that can be harmful.

Ongoing inflammation of the arteries, for example, makes the plaque grow, makes the blood "thick" and contributes to hypertension and possibly to a complete blockage. It is really important to help the body carry out repair of the arteries to its completion, which means to help it replace hard, plaque-laden artery tissue with new, healthy tissue. When repair is carried out properly, the plaque eventually sloughs off and the newly-repaired artery tissue is flexible. This would help reverse hypertension, restore circulation and prevent a heart attack or a stroke.

The reason CVD is so prevalent is that the needed repair doesn't happen properly in so many people. Why is it that in so many people the body is unable to replace damaged artery tissue with new healthy artery tissue?

It is simply because there is recurrent daily damage to the arteries from sticky sugar and from oxidizing seed oils. The body doesn't have enough "raw material" to repair the damage.

A similar process occurs with a scrape or a cut to the skin. The body replaces damaged, scraped or cut skin tissue with new tissue. A scab is formed, and as the healing occurs, the scab sloughs off. The difference between the skin and the arteries is that the skin is left alone to heal. We don't interfere with the healing of the skin by scraping it over and over again or by smearing sugary foods and seed oils on it.

I am providing the healing of the skin as an example because the healing process (inflammation) of both the arteries and the skin is similar: they are both made of the same "stuff".

This is really important to know if you want to know how to prevent or reverse plaque in your arteries and if you want to restore flexibility to your arteries.

Both the skin and the arteries are made of two types of "rope-like" protein, called collagen and elastin (though mostly collagen).

In fact, out of all the thousands of types of protein in the body, the most abundant protein (25% to 30% of the protein mass) is collagen. It is also present in our bones, tendons, ligaments, etc. It provides structure to the body.

While, like any protein, collagen is made of various amino acids, its production is dependent solely on three "ingredients", the amino acids lysine and proline, and vitamin C.

The body uses its reserves of lysine, proline and vitamin C to heal the skin and the arteries. It can usually heal a wound on the skin because there is no interference with the healing. However, it doesn't have enough lysine, proline and vitamin C to repair the arteries because of the recurrent daily damage I mentioned before. So, providing the body with adequate amounts of these building blocks of collagen is really important for the reversal of CVD and I will discuss this idea in more detail in Chapter Ten.

Another important note about inflammation is that it often affects more than just the arteries. Often people with cardiovascular disease also experience inflammation and pain of the joints, known as osteoarthritis. If you experience joint pain, beware of the long-term ingestion of common painkillers (also known as non-steroidal anti-inflammatory drugs), such as lumiracoxib, ibuprofen (Advil), etoricoxib, diclofenac and Celebrex. A review published in the *British Medical Journal* in January 2011 stated that these medications double and triple the risk of heart attack and stroke.[74]

Following the nutritional strategies outlined in Chapter Nine and Chapter Ten will help you reduce your doses or completely eliminate the need for some or all of these medications and your heart medications.

CHAPTER 9

THE HEALTHY HEART DIET

Choosing to follow a heart-healthy diet is essential not only for the prevention of CVD, but also for lasting recovery.

Eating right will do two things. First, it will help stop the damage, the harm that has been done so far (glycation, oxidation and inflammation). Second, eating a healthy diet will allow your body to recover.

The following dietary guidelines are also helpful for weight loss, as well as conditions of inflammation other than cardiovascular disease, such as arthritis, skin and intestinal inflammation, etc.

In this chapter I will discuss each food group – carbohydrates, fats and proteins – as well as healthy snack options and fluid intake.

Carbohydrates

Carbohydrates, primarily glucose and fructose, constitute a source of energy for the body. However, to generate energy from glucose and fructose, certain vitamins and minerals are required. Without nutrients such as certain B vitamins, manganese, magnesium, zinc, copper and others, carbohydrates aren't able to provide energy and they can turn harmful (they contribute to glycation, fat accumulation etc.). Fruit and veggies are healthy because they have lots of nutrients. Baked goods, sweets, candy bars, soda pops and similar foods are harmful because they have almost no beneficial nutrients.

The best sources of carbohydrates
The best carbohydrates we can eat are ones that are high in easily accessible vitamins and minerals. Your primary source of carbohydrates should be fruit and veggies. Enjoy plenty of fruit – tropical, berries and others in that order of preference. Also enjoy real 100% fruit juice (not from concentrate; it is best to make your own fresh juices). Have a fruit and veggie with each meal. Use a fruit as a snack when you want to satisfy a little hunger. Examples of helpful vegetables include carrots, which are great for "sweeping" excess cholesterol out the intestines and celery, which contains a compound called phthalide, which is good for high blood pressure.

Your next best sources of carbohydrates are root vegetables and tubers such as potatoes, yams, cassava, squash, etc.

Non-gluten containing grains are considered "safe" as well; however, the density and availability of their vitamins and minerals is secondary to fruits and vegetables. These include grains such as rice, buck wheat, quinoa, millet, sorghum, teff and corn (although most corn in North America is genetically modified, which poses another concern). Below I include a discussion regarding health concerns about grains.

Carbohydrates to avoid

You may have heard the term "empty calories" before. This refers to any processed food that is devoid of vitamins and minerals. In the Western world we have eaten empty calorie foods for many decades now, especially in the form of refined carbohydrates. In my opinion, this is a problem that has contributed to all the chronic diseases that have plagued us. Carbs and sweeteners that I recommend you avoid completely include anything that contains high fructose corn syrup and any baked product, especially anything made of wheat, (read more on this further below).

Carb sources you should limit include:

- *Baked goods* such as bread (including whole wheat, "whole grain"), pastry, breakfast cereals, pizza and pasta

- *Sweets* including candy and candy bars, ice cream, cookies, cakes and other pastry

- *Soft drinks (soda drinks) and commercially made pasteurized juice.* However, freshly squeezed juice is fine.

- *Sweeteners* such as Splenda (sucralose) and aspartame should be avoided (the safety issues of these chemicals are beyond the scope of this book).

Special notes about grains (especially wheat)

Notice I recommend avoiding wheat as much as possible. This is the most common grain and so I will start my discussion of grains with wheat.

The commonly-used variety of wheat in North America, called Dwarf Wheat, is high in a starch called amylopectin A, which is "very starchy". There is no difference whether you eat white bread or whole grain bread, the impact on your blood sugar levels from the starch in wheat is the same. Daily consumption of bread and other starchy foods that are devoid of vitamins and minerals can lead to atherosclerosis and insulin resistance.

Many readers will likely benefit from restricting wheat and other gluten-containing grains for another reason – the presence of gluten. Other grains that contain this protein include rye, barley and spelt. Gliadin, a molecule which is a part of gluten, causes tiny microscopic gaps (tears) in the intestinal wall, which result in the "leakage" of sometimes undesired

65

substances through these gaps into the circulation. This can lead to various immune and inflammatory conditions, such as skin rashes, digestive issues, sinus and respiratory issues and even on-going anxiety (which can affect blood pressure). I had several clients who suffered from anxiety until they decided to give up all gluten containing grains (and sometimes all grains).

If you choose to continue eating bread and grains, perhaps you could choose bread made of sprouted grains and breads made of fermented flour (sour dough) as these contain less gluten. Just try to limit the quantity you eat. You could also try specialty crackers with high fiber content. Such crackers weigh less, but due to the fiber content will satisfy your hunger with only a few pieces.

Sweeteners
North Americans use an average of more than twenty-two teaspoons of sugar a day. Most of it comes from processed foods and sweetened beverages. There is nothing wrong with consuming a few teaspoons of sugar each day (added to your coffee or to other food) if your overall diet is healthy. In fact, it is beneficial to sweeten your coffee with a little bit of sugar in order to avoid hypoglycemia. However, there are safe sugar alternatives that help limit the daily intake of refined sugar.

Enjoy moderate amounts of raw honey, which is relatively rich in nutrients needed to turn the sugar in honey into energy.

Stevia is a non-sugar containing safe sweetener. It is a powder extracted from the leaves of the plant stevia rebaudiana, which is up to 300 times sweeter than sugar. However, its sweetness comes from substances called steviol glycosides, not from its glucose or fructose content. Not only does this make stevia a safe sweetener, some studies have shown it to be beneficial for diabetics.

Other safe sweeteners include sugar alcohols such as xylitol and erythritol. These sweet compounds are only partially absorbed by the intestines. They are safe and cause no rise in blood sugar levels. In high amounts they could cause some gas and maybe diarrhea, but this shouldn't be the case when used at less than 65g/day (one teaspoon holds 5g).

Oils and fats

Next to water, which makes up about 60% of the human body, fat is the next most common substance. Unless obese, the fat content of men is generally between 14% and 24% and of women is between 21% and 31%. I believe that daily intake of fat should be between 25% and 35% of total daily caloric intake. Having said that, when you look at the fat intake of healthy indigenous societies throughout the world, fat consumption varies from a few percentage points to as high as 70% (the traditional Arctic Inuit diet and the diet of the Masai tribe in Africa). The reason they have no evidence of heart disease is that they consume lots of saturated fat and relatively small amount of polyunsaturated oils, and that is the key. The key is to consume the right kind of fat.

Good oils

As you read in Chapter Four, saturated fat and, to a lesser extent, monounsaturated fat, are the fats of choice for health, while polyunsaturated fat is what you need to limit.

For cooking, use coconut oil, butter, palm kernel oil and beef tallow.

For salad dressings, use (sparingly) some olive oil or avocado oil (high in monounsaturated fatty acids).

Your saturated fat will typically come from dairy products (including milk, cream butter and cheese), eggs, poultry, meat and coconut oil.

Avoid polyunsaturated oils and their derivatives

Since there are some polyunsaturated oils in most foods, you will get some in. However in order to keep the amount of polyunsaturated oils to a minimum, avoid cooking with most plant oils (canola, soy, corn, cottonseed, sunflower seed safflower, and grape seed oil). Also, lots of different commercially prepared foods, including salad dressings and dips, contain vegetable oils.

To avoid trans fatty acids and hydrogenated oils, you need to read labels. Labels on foods containing trans fats may describe their ingredients as hydrogenated or partially hydrogenated fat, as well as "interesterified" fat. In the fast food industry, the oils used in deep frying typically have trans fats.

Common foods containing trans fatty acids and hydrogenated oils include margarine, packaged baked goods (including breakfast cereals), and frozen goods such as pizza, pies, and fish sticks.

Protein

The daily requirement of protein is about 0.8g per kg of body weight for a sedentary or mildly active person, which translates to about 0.36g per pound of body weight. However, if you have no kidney disease you can safely take up to two times that amount. Generally, the more physically active you are, the more you need. Other sources suggest the average female should consume 80g a day and the average male consume 100g a day. Getting an adequate amount of protein is important for optimal health. Having said that, there are societies in the world that subsist on far less protein and are still free of chronic disease such as CVD. Choose protein sources that are as unprocessed as possible. So avoid stuff like luncheon meats, microwave dinners and, in general, read labels to avoid unhealthy preservatives, additives, sweeteners and artificial colors and flavors.

Proteins represent the trickiest food group to make general statements about because most food allergies and sensitivities people may experience are associated with different types of proteins. Even gluten, while it comes from wheat and other grains, is essentially a protein. Some people don't do well with casein, a milk protein, others may react to one of the proteins in eggs, etc. So, while the information I present here is general, don't eat anything I recommend if you are allergic or sensitive to it.

I believe the best sources of protein to be organic milk and certain dairy products, free range eggs and collagen-containing structures from meat and poultry (skin, cartilage, bones – can be used in soups). These sources of protein have a well-balanced amino acid profile (amino acids are the building blocks of protein). Milk also offers the benefit of providing some naturally occurring sugar and a good proportion of saturated fat, while eggs and cheese, in additional to the protein, also offer good healthy saturated and monounsaturated fat.

Dairy products

While milk and dairy products provide potentially high-quality nourishment, sensitivities or allergies to milk, including lactose intolerance, are some of the most common food allergies. I don't share the view of many natural health practitioners that there is inherently anything wrong with milk itself. I believe that most of the allergies and sensitivities that milk may cause are associated with what the cows consume (in their feed, etc.), with its production process (pasteurization) and with the additives added to dairy products.

Regarding lactose intolerance, according to Dr. Ray Peat (www.raypeat.com), the difficulty in digesting lactose (milk sugar) stems from the effect of factors such as endotoxins produced by "unfriendly" intestinal bacterial, hypothyroidism and low progesterone levels. All these factors diminish the amount of available lactase enzyme in the intestines (the enzyme responsible for producing lactose). One study showed that when people with lactose intolerance were given a small amount of milk daily, they were able to adapt and tolerate lactose much better[75].

In the US, dairy cows are fed growth hormones to maximize milk production and in both the US and Canada, they are fed antibiotics. Both of these substances end up in the milk supply. Pesticides and herbicides in the cows' feed also end up in the milk and can be potentially be harmful.

Pasteurization, the heating up of milk to kill any disease causing microbes, is another concern. It alters the shape of one of the types of protein in milk. The main types of protein in milk are casein (82%) and two kinds of whey globulins – alpha and beta (18%). While casein is fairly resilient to heat, the shape of the whey globulins is altered by heat[76]. Changes to the shape of a food protein can potentially make it harmful (an allergen). Based on the incidence of reported food-borne illnesses, I believe raw, or non-pasteurized dairy is safer than leafy greens for human consumption, but as it stands, it is not widely available for people living in North America.

The last issue is the addition of thickening agents (carrageenan, guar gum, xanthan gum, corn starch, and perhaps other agents) and artificial food coloring to certain dairy products. These substances can lead to allergies and potentially be harmful to human health, but the average consumer may sometimes erroneously, attribute any reactions he or she may observe to the dairy milk itself.

In the absence of raw dairy products, I believe that organic dairy products are generally safe and nutritious. The feed used in organic dairy farming is devoid of pesticides, herbicides and antibiotics. As well, organic dairy products are generally devoid of potentially harmful additives. Your products should only include bacterial culture, microbial enzymes or rennet and perhaps added nutrients such as vitamin D.

Allergies and sensitivities to dairy can manifest as gastrointestinal discomfort, skin rashes and respiratory issues. If you think that dairy may be causing any health problems for you, just discontinue it for a week or two and see if these health problems improve.

Eggs

Eggs offer 6g of protein per serving and offer lots of good nutrients. I prefer eggs from organic, free range chickens because they tend to offer more nutrients, including vitamin E and A.[77] I have no problem supporting consumption of as many eggs as you'd like or tolerate daily.

Not only can you benefit from the egg white and egg yolk, the shell also offers a unique nutritional value. It is rich in calcium and other minerals. One whole medium sized eggshell makes about one teaspoon of powder, which yields about 750 – 800 mgs of elemental calcium plus other microelements such as magnesium, boron, copper, iron, manganese, molybdenum, sulfur, silicon, zinc, etc. You can grind washed and air-dried egg shells in a coffee grinder, store it and take ½ tea spoon with food once or twice a day.

Meat and poultry

These sources can easily provide you with all or most of your daily protein requirements in one meal as they contain an average of 20% or more of protein by weight. However, ideally you should consume them with the skin and cartilage, which are rich in collagen. Bone broth soups can also help provide some gelatin (broken collagen) and could benefit you, especially if you have CVD, arthritis and related conditions.

Fish and seafood

To minimize exposure to antibiotics and hormones, fish and seafood should be "wild" (from oceans and lakes), not farmed. However, even wild fish contains contaminants in the form of heavy metals that pollute the oceans. Therefore, it is recommended to eat fish only two to three times a week. Small fish concentrate fewer toxins in their bodies than large fish.

Beans and lentils

Beans and lentils should be soaked for six to twenty-four hours with 1-2 tbsp of vinegar or lemon juice and drained before you cook them in order to minimize the consumption of a harmful group of substances called lectins and phytates. Canned beans should be rinsed well. They contain about 10% protein, depending on the type of bean.

Nuts and seeds

While they offer a fair amount of protein, I would use them as a snack, not as a primary source of protein, because they also contain lots of polyunsaturated oils.

Conversely, they also contain healthy nutrients, including antioxidants that can potentially protect against any damage from the polyunsaturated oils. It is better to eat them raw and not roasted. They are even more nutritious when you soak them in water for a few minutes, drain the water and leave them in the fridge overnight. This initiates sprouting, which makes the vitamins and minerals more bio-available. Pre-packaged nuts and seeds are usually roasted with vegetable oils. Some are sold as dry roasted (baked). You could also roast or bake them yourself in the oven.

Snacks

Enjoy fruit, nuts and seeds, mix into your plain yogurt some fruit and enjoy some dark chocolate. Snack on veggies as well, and find ways to make them more palatable by using dips such as hummus (made of pureed chick pea and sesame seeds) or certain dairy-based dips. You can also get a vegetable dehydrator and turn your veggies into healthy chips. Look for desserts that are made from coca, coconut and natural healthy sweeteners.

Water and liquids

It is popular to think that we need eight cups of water a day. However, remember that most food contains about 60%-70% water. So let your thirst guide you. I like starting my day with one or two cups of water with squeezed lemon, which I find quite refreshing.

Drink clean filtered or spring water from a reliable source. If your water is distilled, make sure to add some trace minerals to it. You can get liquid preparations of trace minerals from health stores.

Try to avoid unfiltered tap water that contains chlorine and fluoride. Fluoride is implicated in collagen degeneration, which can lead to osteoporosis, osteoarthritis and CVD.

If you are a coffee drinker, limit your intake to one to two cups a day. Dark roast has less caffeine. Add a little sugar or honey to avoid hypoglycemia.

I also recommend that you explore various therapeutic herbal teas. For example, fennel tea for digestion, hawthorn tea for cardiovascular support, etc.

Salt

Since most salt in an average North American diet is consumed from processed foods, when you start eating healthy you will likely get less salt. In general, if you stay away from food with added sodium, it is a good idea to add about a teaspoon and a half of salt to your diet every day. You can sprinkle it on food throughout the day or you can add some to juice or water. This will allow you to get a sufficient amount of sodium and any excess will be eliminated by the kidneys. If this sounds too high to you, review the information in Chapter Five. As long as you are consuming enough potassium (see next chapter), these levels of sodium will not harm you; in fact, you will benefit from it.

The DASH diet?

My guidelines are somewhat more demanding than the principles of the DASH diet. DASH is an acronym that stands for Dietary Approaches to Stop Hypertension. This diet is as beneficial as medications for lowering blood pressure![78]

The DASH guidelines are somewhat more lenient than my recommendations, mostly in terms of allowing grains. However, my clinical experience has shown me that limiting grains in your diet in favor of fruit and veggies is necessary in order to normalize blood pressure, heal cardiovascular disease and even lose weight.

Mindful eating

The last piece I want to leave you with in this chapter is the difference between "living to eat" versus "eating to live". Overeating can't be healthy. Eat when you are hungry. Become more mindful of why you eat at any given moment and pay attention to your thirst level. Sometimes we eat when we are actually thirsty.

Chew your food well and don't rush when you eat. If you experience digestive discomfort after you eat, try to discern whether a certain food didn't "agree" with you, then eliminate it for a while and see if digestion becomes better. You can seek the assistance of a healthcare practitioner to discern if you have any allergies or sensitivities to food. You could also test out the use of digestive enzymes from a health store or a pharmacy to improve your digestion.

Try to avoid proton pump inhibitors, medications used to treat "acid reflux", as studies show that they can do more harm than good in the long run. They are associated with decreased bone density and increased risk of fractures.[79] Common brand names of such medications include Pariet, Nexium and Losec, and their general names end with the suffix "prazole", as in (omeprazole, etc.).

Listen to your body to discern if your desire to eat is sometimes driven by your emotions. In that case integrating modalities such as counselling or means to reduce stress could be helpful. I will discuss stress management and aspects of mind-body medicine in Chapter Eleven.

As you follow my dietary guidelines, you will be well nourished without experiencing hunger.

A naturopathic doctor, a holistic nutritionist or other qualified health practitioners can assess your health and guide you with suggestions that are specifically tailored to your needs.

In Doctor Klein's Healthy Heart Seminar (*www.drkleinhealthyheart.com*), I walk clients through activities and exercises that enable them to construct individualized, easy-to-follow meal plans.

CHAPTER 10

LET THY VITAMINS BE THY MEDICINE

Why Vitamins and Minerals Are Good for You

What are vitamins and minerals for?

Many studies have demonstrated the benefits of different nutrients in improving blood pressure, normalizing blood lipids, preventing heart attacks and strokes and even reversing plaque in the arteries.

There is a general acceptance that vitamins and minerals are "good for you". But what does that mean?

Vitamins and minerals are simply the necessary tools your body requires to assemble or disassemble important substances for your wellbeing. These substances can be different enzymes, hormones, proteins, structures within your cells or outside your cells, etc. Vitamins are simply necessary for life.

For example, in an earlier chapter I explained how the sugar you eat is used to generate energy. Sugar can be disassembled and processed to generate energy only if certain vitamins and minerals, such as vitamins B2 and B3 (and other B vitamins), manganese and magnesium, are available as tools to facilitate the process.

While all the nutrients discussed in this chapter naturally occur in food, it is often difficult – and sometimes impossible – to get sufficient amounts for restoration of health from our diet alone. Modern-day agricultural practices have depleted the amount of nutrients in the soil and, as a result, the produce we eat isn't as rich in nutrients as it used to be.

Supplementation can speed up recovery and is certainly needed for individuals who don't follow a heart-healthy diet. When one follows a healthy diet, most supplemental vitamins and minerals are needed only for a limited period of time.

Consult a naturopathic doctor, a qualified health practitioner or an experienced nutritionist to help you select the right supplements and dosages for your needs.

A novel approach by a Nobel Prize scientist

Before I introduce you to the most relevant vitamins and minerals for cardiovascular well-being, I would like to introduce you to what is, in my mind, the most powerful and yet simple approach to reversing plaque.

This approach was developed by a two-time Nobel recipient, the late Dr. Linus Pauling, and by Dr. Mathias Rath. In fact, in 1991 they registered a patent on a formulation they developed for the treatment of "occlusive heart disease" (in other words, for reversing plaque in the arteries) and for inhibiting lipoprotein A (a lipoprotein they believed was involved in laying down plaque).[80]

The formulation consisted of both pharmaceutical substances and natural agents. The pharmaceutical component dealt mostly with lipoprotein A, while the natural component dealt with the reversal of the plaque itself.

In the chapter on inflammation and repair, I established that the body attempts to repair any damaged or injured tissue, including the arteries. However, due to the constant damage from glycation, oxidation and on-going inflammation, the body may not have enough of the raw materials it requires to replace old, sticky and hardened arterial collagen and elastin with healthy collagen and elastin.

Dr. Pauling and Dr. Rath knew that two key amino acids and a vitamin were required for the production of collagen. These were lysine, proline and vitamin C. Without sufficient amounts of these key substances, the body can't produce enough collagen and elastin to repair the arteries.

Drs. Pauling and Rath realized that in order to help the body repair its arteries, it is important to supplement with sufficient amounts of lysine, proline and vitamin C. As the arteries get repaired, the arterial plaque, much like a scab on a healing scrape or cut to the skin, gradually sloughs off. When I explain this to people, some are concerned that plaque can dislodge and cause a blockage. However, plaque doesn't dislodge all at once, it sloughs off gradually. The minute plaque particles are carried to the liver, into the bile duct, which empties into the intestines, and are then eliminated by the colon.

Dr. Pauling published the results of his early experiments with his novel approach in two scientific journals.[81, 82, 83] He made recommendations to a few individuals who had a history of angina (chest pain due to advanced blockages in the coronary arteries). He suggested they consume daily between 5g to 6g of lysine and vitamin C in divided doses. These individuals reported complete alleviation of the chest pain and improved circulation and activity levels within a few short weeks of starting the regimen.

In 1994, Dr. Rath and a colleague, Dr. Niedzwiecki, PhD, conducted a clinical trial on 55 individuals with various stages of coronary artery disease (presence of plaque).[84] For the first six months, they just monitored the rate of plaque growth. They noted that in subjects with more advanced coronary artery disease the plaque grew at a faster rate than in those with early coronary artery disease. Then the study subjects were instructed to take a nutritional formulation consisting of lysine (450mg), proline (450mg) and vitamin C (2700mg), with additional beneficial vitamins and minerals, for another twelve months. At the end of the twelve months, changes in plaque deposition were assessed. Results ranged from complete halting of plaque deposition to complete disappearance of plaque in some subjects!

In my experience, effective dosages of these nutrients would range from 2g-6g of lysine and vitamin C and 1g-2g of proline. The amount taken would depend on whether you follow a heart-healthy diet based on the guidelines outlined in the previous chapter. More lysine may be required than proline because lysine is an essential nutrient (the body doesn't produce it on it own), whereas proline is non-essential (it is produced by the body to a certain extent).

This approach is also helpful to many who have high blood pressure because as the arteries are repaired they become elastic (flexible) again. As flexibility is restored, blood pressure improves, too. In my experience, this approach often results in improvement in blood pressure and overall circulation within weeks. Other benefits of assisting with the body's production and repair of collagen include: improvement in bone strength, reduced joint inflammation, improvement in skin tone, etc.

Other important nutrients

Other nutrients play important roles in the prevention and treatment of cardiovascular disease.

The first four nutrients (and class of nutrients) listed below are, in my mind, the most important ones, particularly because they are the ones we are most deficient in.

Vitamin C

This well-known vitamin is often taken for granted.

Because of its role in repairing the arteries and reversing plaque, vitamin C has been shown to be important in preventing strokes and heart attacks. Vitamin C is an important antioxidant, which means it helps to protect against oxidation. It doesn't just help protect against oxidation of the arteries, it also helps prevent the oxidation of cholesterol.

Studies have found vitamin C helpful at lowering blood pressure and normalizing cholesterol. In one study, individuals who consumed 500mg of vitamin C daily had an average reduction in systolic blood pressure (upper number) of 9% over one month.[85] In 1985, scientists showed in a lab that vitamin C also helped to inhibit the activity of Co HMG reductase (a key enzyme responsible for producing cholesterol) and concluded that vitamin C may be required for regulation of cholesterol production.[86]

Vitamin C helps control cholesterol levels in another way. Cholesterol is eliminated through the intestines after it is converted to bile acid. Vitamin C is needed for this conversion.[87] Some research suggests that vitamin C may have a normalizing effect on cholesterol and triglycerides at levels of 1000mg and higher.[88]

Vitamin C and cardiovascular disease

A landmark 1992 study of over 11,000 individuals who took 300mg vitamin C daily showed a 42% reduction in deaths from cardiovascular disease in men and a 25% reduction in women. As well, those who took 300mg vitamin C a day lived six years longer.[89]

According to a twenty-year-long Japanese study published in the medical journal *Stroke* in October 2000, vitamin C was the single most important factor in preventing strokes.[90]

While dietary sources of vitamin C are important, I recommend supplementing with at least 1000mg to 2000mg a day for optimal health and prevention of cardiovascular disease. Dietary sources of vitamin C include: guava (1/2 cup, 188mg), red pepper (1/2 cup, 142mg), kiwi and orange (1 medium, 70mg) and grapefruit juice (1 cup, 50mg-70mg), as well as many other fruits and vegetables.

The FDA maintains that getting less than 100mg of vitamin C a day is all you need. However, many vitamin C researchers explain that while the FDA recommended daily allowance is sufficient to prevent scurvy, it is not sufficient for the treatment of health conditions that require vitamin C (CVD, osteoarthritis, osteoporosis, certain cancers, etc). Therefore, in order to reverse cardiovascular disease, particularly if you want to remove plaque from your arteries, you'd likely benefit from taking, at the very least, upwards of 2000g a day for a period of six to eighteen months (along with the amino acid lysine and, to a lesser extent, the amino acid proline). Some vitamin C advocates take about 10,000mg daily.

High amounts of vitamin C should be taken in divided doses.

A note of caution regarding vitamin C
Continuous intake of high amounts of this beneficial vitamin can deplete copper and manganese from your body. These are trace minerals, a term that describes minerals that are needed in trace amounts. Good food sources of manganese are pineapple, brown rice, garbanzo beans and spinach. Good food sources of copper are calf liver and crimini mushrooms, as well as nuts and seeds (a few Brazil nuts can provide plenty of copper), vegetables and legumes. A general good source of trace minerals is seaweed. You can also get trace mineral supplements.

Some people have various degrees of allergies to vitamin C, particularly to ascorbic acid, the metabolically active form. Some of those individuals do well with vitamin C supplements derived from plant sources, such as acerola or camu camu.

Vitamin C and iron absorption
Vitamin C also increases iron absorption, which can be helpful for people who have iron deficiency anemia. However, if you know that you have hemochromatosis, a condition of elevated iron levels, you ought to be cautious and seek medical advice.

Vitamin C and kidney stones

Doctors may be concerned that high amounts of vitamin C cause kidney stones. However, most large-scale research has shown no formation of kidney stones.[91, 92, 93, 94] The highest amount of vitamin C tested was 2000mg (2g). To prevent kidney stone formation, make sure to drink a sufficient amount of water and avoid foods that cause loss of calcium, such as ... you guessed it, refined carbohydrates and polyunsaturated oils. Eating vegetables also helps to protect against kidney stones.

Magnesium

Magnesium is an extremely important mineral. It is involved in more than three hundred metabolic processes in the body. Studies show that a significant portion of people with high blood pressure and diabetes are low in magnesium.

Taking magnesium has shown to help lower blood pressure.[95] Magnesium does this in several ways. Magnesium is necessary for relaxing the muscles. Since the arteries are lined by muscle cells, lack of magnesium may cause them to contract, which may constrict the arteries. Magnesium ensures the arteries stay relaxed and dilated.[96]

Magnesium is the most important nutrient for the management of stress and anxiety. It is necessary for the production of important neurotransmitters (messenger molecules) in the nervous system, including acetylcholine, a neurotransmitter responsible for overall relaxation.

Magnesium helps prevent and reverse oxidation and, therefore, inflammation. As such, it is helpful in the healing process of the arteries.

Magnesium also acts as a natural statin (cholesterol-lowering drug). As you know from the information presented in Chapter Three, statin drugs block a key enzyme responsible for producing cholesterol called Co HmG reductase. Magnesium is a natural deactivator of this enzyme. Low magnesium levels will likely increase the production of this enzyme. In addition to normalizing LDL cholesterol, magnesium helps increase HDL cholesterol and lower triglycerides.[97]

How do you know if you are deficient in magnesium?

Magnesium deficiency can be detected by doing a blood test. A common magnesium blood test is one that measures magnesium in the plasma (blood fluid). However, this test is only good for detecting an extreme deficiency of magnesium. A better test is one that measures the magnesium levels of red blood cells.

However, you can detect magnesium deficiency by the presence of signs and symptoms related to or caused by magnesium deficiency. Common signs of deficiency include headaches, poor sleep, muscle cramps, restless leg syndrome and anxiety. Supplementing with a good source and the correct dose of magnesium would likely improve and possibly eliminate these conditions.

It is almost certain that individuals with high blood pressure and diabetes, as well as other conditions such as arrhythmia (irregular heart beat), arthritis and myalgia (muscle pain) and constipation, likely have insufficient magnesium.

The recommended daily intake of magnesium is 320mg for an adult female and 420mg for an adult male. In a state of deficiency, more may be required. You can use magnesium supplements to resolve magnesium deficiency. These supplements come in various forms, such as magnesium citrate, magnesium glucantate, magnesium chloride, magnesium bisglycinate, etc. Certain factors such as advanced age and poor digestive health can limit absorption of magnesium (and other minerals). In my experience, for better absorption use magnesium chloride or magnesium glycinate or a supplement that offers free magnesium ions, in which case a lower dose (25mg-50mg) is sufficient.

Dietary sources of magnesium include non-processed oat bran and buckwheat, which offer some of the highest amounts of magnesium (200-300mg per cup), along with squash, pumpkin, sun flower and sesame seeds, cocoa powder (dark chocolate), seaweed, legumes (beans and lentils), fish and green leafy vegetables such as spinach.

Iodine
Iodine is a mineral necessary for the production of thyroid hormone.

People who have low thyroid hormone levels (hypothyroidism) are more prone to developing plaque in the arteries and have higher blood pressure levels.[98] Common symptoms of hypothyroidism are: low energy levels, difficulty losing weight, low basal temperature (feeling cold), mental slowness or "fogginess", predisposition to depression, poor sleep, a slow pulse, thinning hair and weak nails, dry skin, constipation and slight puffiness due to water retention. Prolonged deficiency can cause a goiter, which is an enlarged thyroid gland.

When doctors recognize these symptoms they normally order a blood test to measure thyroid hormone levels and thyroid stimulating hormone (TSH). Doctors would normally diagnose hypothyroidism if the blood test indicates so. However, often when blood test results appear normal and symptoms of hypothyroidism still exist, it is likely that the condition is real as well.

Causes of hypothyroidism include deficiency of iodine; consuming too much chlorine and fluorine, which diminishes iodine absorption (usually from municipal drinking water); suppression of the thyroid gland by polyunsaturated oils (vegetable oils); and the presence of high insulin and estrogen. The thyroid gland, located in the front of the neck, requires 70micrograms of iodine a day to make the thyroid hormone. It produces the less active form of the hormone, T4, which travels to the liver where it is converted to the active form, T3, with the assistance of the trace mineral selenium. The recommended daily intake of iodine is about 150 micrograms a day, more for pregnant and nursing women. Some doctors, including me, believe it is perfectly safe and often desirable to consume iodine at levels that are several times higher than the recommended daily intake.

The best dietary source of iodine is seaweed (kelp).

Optimizing iodine consumption can be done by eating seaweed or, better yet, by drinking its juice or liquid extract. This will help improve production of the thyroid hormone.

Potassium

This mineral is necessary for regulating blood pressure and regulating the electric impulses in the heart, which control the contraction and relaxation of the heart (heart beat and heart rate). The recommended daily intake is 3500mg.

A diet rich in fruit, vegetables and good-quality protein has plenty of potassium. People who eat refined and processed foods and those who are taking potassium-depleting diuretic medications run the risk of being deficient in potassium.

Potassium-depleting diuretics consist of three groups of medications: thiazide diuretics, loop diuretics and carbonic anhydrase inhibitors. If you are on diuretics, ask your doctor or pharmacist or consult the Internet to determine if it is the potassium-depleting kind.

Moderately low levels of potassium may be associated with high blood pressure and increased risk for CVD, especially stroke.[99] Severe deficiency, as with magnesium, is associated with greater risk of arrhythmia (irregular heart rate). Because of the role of potassium in sugar uptake by the cells, its deficiency may also contribute to diabetes.

In certain jurisdictions the dose in over-the-counter potassium supplements is limited to less than 100mg and a doctor's prescription may be needed (check in with your local health store and pharmacy to find out). However, a wholesome Healthy Heart diet, the kind I describe in this book, should provide you with plenty of potassium.

Excess potassium levels are not common, but can indicate kidney disease or an adrenal gland disease called Addison's disease. In such cases there needs to be a controlled consumption of potassium rich foods.

Co Enzyme Q10

Co enzyme Q10 is a substance the body makes for the purpose of assisting in producing energy in our cells. The heart, which never stops beating, harbors some of the highest levels of Co enzyme Q10. People who experience heart failure or cardiomyopathy tend to have low levels of Co enzyme Q10, so their hearts are too weak and can't pump blood properly. Studies show that Co enzyme Q10 supplementation is helpful in improving recovery from a heart attack and preventing recurrence of a heart attack. [100, 101] It can also help stabilize an irregular heart-beat, improve congestive heart failure and lower high blood pressure. [102, 103]

The human body utilizes vitamins C, certain B vitamins, magnesium, selenium and the amino acid tyrosine to produce Co enzyme Q10. You can also get Co enzyme Q10 from your diet. Food sources that are richest in Co enzyme Q10 are fish and organ meats (liver, kidney) and germ of whole grains. Liver and kidney contain 2mg-3mg of Co enzyme Q10 per ounce, while whole grain germ provides less.

Food sources, while valuable, may not provide adequate amounts of Co enzyme Q10 to individuals who have cardiovascular disease. Supplementation may then be warranted. While therapeutic doses start at 30mg a day, most studies that showed positive results used at least 60mg per day. Even higher doses (between 60mg to 200mg) may be required for individuals who take medications that deplete CoQ10 levels in the body. These medications include statin drugs, beta blockers, thiazide diuretics, a class of diabetic medications called sulfonylureas, a class of antidepressants called tricyclic antidepressants and a few others.

Antioxidants

Next I will discuss the role of some key antioxidants. Any substance that can counter oxidation (bind an electron) is considered an antioxidant. The antioxidants most fundamental to human health are *vitamin C, vitamin E, selenium, and vitamin A* (made from beta carotenes). In addition to being antioxidants, these nutrients play other necessary biological roles, so these are really important.

Antioxidants counter oxidation, thereby assisting in the prevention and reversal of arterial plaque and inflammation. Dr. Pauling and Dr. Rath included vitamin E and beta carotenes in their original formulation.[104]

Vitamin A

Beta carotenes belong to a class of nutrients called carotenoids. Beta carotene and some carotenoids are made into vitamin A. Vitamin A constitutes a group of several closely-related substances, all with important roles to play in the body and all with antioxidant properties.

Many studies show that a diet rich in beta carotenes (fruit and vegetables) protects against cardiovascular disease. However, according to my research, most studies failed to conclude that beta carotene *supplements* have a direct impact on reducing plaque in the arteries.

One important function of vitamin A is its assistance (along with T3, the active form of the thyroid hormone) in converting cholesterol to various important steroid hormones, such as pregnenolone, progesterone and DHEA. As such, it helps prevent the accumulation of excessive amounts of cholesterol and reverse other conditions related to excessive estrogen.

Since vitamin A is a fat soluble vitamin, dietary sources of this vitamin include dairy products (including butter), eggs, fish oil (including the well-known cod liver oil) and organ meats. These are the type of foods avoided by those who follow a conventional "cardio protective" diet. However, the lack of vitamin A, paradoxically, can cause elevation of cholesterol levels. It can be produced by carotenes, but that production is limited in diabetics, people with hypothyroidism and those with diseases of the digestive system.

The daily recommended intake for this vitamin is 700mcg (2300IU) – 900mcg (3000IU). However, more could be better for people with CVD and related health issues. Vitamin A should not be taken at more than 15,000IU by anyone with liver disease. Otherwise, up to 25,000IU a day of vitamin A would be well tolerated by most. Vitamin A can be used at higher levels to treat specific conditions, but only under medical supervision. The most common supplemental sources of vitamin A include multivitamins and cod liver oil. Generally, daily inclusion of vitamin A dietary sources should provide enough vitamin A.

Vitamin E

Vitamin E, another fat soluble vitamin, has been shown in several large studies to be a protective nutrient. For example, in the two studies referenced here, it lowered the risk of heart attack by 34% in women[105] and by 40% in men.[106]

Regarding vitamin E supplements, you should consider that vitamin E refers not to one single substance, but to a group of substance called tocopherols. They come as alpha, beta, gamma and delta tocopherols. It is believed that all of them play a role in countering oxidation; however, most studies to date on supplementing with vitamin E have been carried out with the alpha form only. The alpha form can come as a natural or a "d" alpha tocopherol, or as a synthetic form "dl" alpha tocopherol. Based on the current data, the natural form is more active than the synthetic form (which is more common in vitamin E supplements) by 33% to 50%. If you use vitamin E supplements or use a nutritional formulation containing vitamin E, try to get one that has the natural alpha form or one with a mixture of several forms.

Food sources high in vitamin E are sunflower seeds, almonds, olives, mustard and turnip greens, spinach, papaya and blueberries. Food sources provide a mixture of tocopherols. The recommended daily intake of vitamin E is 15mg or 22.5 IU. It is generally possible to get sufficient amounts of vitamin E from a healthy diet. Supplemental vitamin E requirements diminish when consumption of polyunsaturated oils is significantly reduced.

Selenium
The trace mineral selenium enhances the antioxidant effect of vitamin E on lipids. While it is not a direct cure, some studies found that deficiency is associated with increased mortality from CVD. Often, supplements containing vitamin E also contain selenium.

Recommended daily intake is 55mcg a day, an amount easily obtained by eating two Brazil nuts a day. Other good sources include fish, sea food, seeds and veggies.

Alpha Lipoic Acid

This is an important antioxidant that is active both in water (water soluble) and fat (fat soluble), making it effective at countering oxidation in all the tissues of the body. It plays an important role in the utilization of sugar to produce energy and is very helpful in managing blood sugar levels, which is important to protect the arteries.

Dosages would range from 600mg to 1800mg. Food sources include meat, liver, brewer's yeast, spinach and broccoli.

Flavonoids

Another important class of dietary antioxidants is flavonoids. This includes many substances that are commonly found in fruit and vegetables (especially the skin) and are particularly high in foods such as berries, citrus fruit, dark chocolate and tea. Flavonoids have been shown to be protective for the cardiovascular system.[107]

B vitamins

There are a number of B vitamins and most of them, if not all, play a direct or an indirect role in protecting your heart and arteries. The vitamins highlighted below are the main ones for treatment of CVD.

Vitamin B3 (niacin)

Vitamin B3 (niacin) has long been established by the PDR (the Physicians' Desk Reference) as a "drug" for lowering LDL cholesterol and triglycerides, increasing HDL and reducing the risk of developing CVD. The therapeutic dose for lowering cholesterol is up to 1500mg-2000mg in divided doses. However, at times liver problems may occur at these levels, so it has to be taken under supervision. Also, levels upwards of 75mg can bring about a "niacin flush". This is an uncomfortable flushing of the skin, accompanied by a sensation of heat and sometimes nausea, which occurs from dilation of the arteries. Niacinamide, another form of this vitamin, doesn't cause the flushing, but it hasn't been shown to be helpful in lowering cholesterol.

To avoid the flushing effect and still derive the benefit, you could use a "slow release" or "sustained release" form of niacin supplements. A study published in the November 2009 issue of the *New England Journal of Medicine* showed reduction in atherosclerosis with 2000mg of the sustained release form of niacin taken for fourteen months.[108]

Vitamins B6, B12 and folic acid
Vitamins B6, B12 and folic acid help to control the amount of circulating homocysteine. Homocysteine is a metabolic by-product which, at high amounts, is considered a significant risk factor for cardiovascular disease. Too much of it can degrade collagen (including arterial collagen), elastin and proteoglycans (another component of connective tissue present in the arteries). In one study, supplementation with this combination of vitamins showed a reduction in plaque.[109]

Vitamin D

In recent years, much information has become available about the importance of vitamin D beyond just bone health.

It is important to ensure adequate levels of vitamin D. A single twenty- to thirty-minute exposure to the sun in the summer (when at least 40% of the body is uncovered) would result in the production of 10,000 to 20,000 international units of vitamin D. This is far more than the current official recommendation of no more than 2000IU daily.

Vitamin D deficiency is related to CVD [110] and hypertension. According to research, vitamin D may lower blood pressure,[111] particularly in those who are deficient in vitamin D.

There is much research on the importance of vitamin D in the prevention and treatment of cardiovascular disease. If you would like to find out more about the importance of vitamin D, not only for cardiovascular health, go the wonderfully resourceful web site of the Vitamin D Council, *www.vitamindcouncil.org*. Based on the recommendations of the council, most healthy adults living in the northern hemisphere, where access to direct sunlight is limited in the fall and winter, would benefit from daily supplementation of at least 5000 IU.

People with these conditions should only take vitamin D with the guidance of a knowledgeable physician: primary hyperparathyroidism, sarcoidosis, granulomatous TB and some cancers.

Calcium

Studies show that insufficient intake of calcium is associated with hypertension.[112],[113] The recommended daily intake of calcium for adults is between 1000mg to 1200mg. A healthy diet should be able to provide the needed daily calcium requirements. Food sources high in calcium include dairy products, sesame seeds, broccoli and green leafy veggies, almonds and sardines. Dietary calcium absorption can be limited by not having enough vitamin D (refer to the brief discussion above about vitamin D).

Vitamin K

The two naturally occurring forms of Vitamin K are K1 and K2. Vitamin K1 is readily available from green leafy vegetables, and is converted in the gut by certain bacteria and in certain organs to vitamin K2. Vitamin K2 is important for reversing the accumulation of calcium in the arteries, a process that contributes to hardening of the plaque material. Adequate levels of vitamin K may prevent plaque calcification and perhaps be a helpful component in reversing calcification.[114],[115]

The daily required intake of 70mcg to 80mcg can be easily obtained from a couple of servings of green leafy vegetables such as salad greens, collard greens, spinach, kale, broccoli, cabbage, etc. To ensure adequate levels of vitamin K2 enjoy small amounts of fermented foods such as kefir, sauerkraut (fermented cabbage), etc.

Herbs

Readers of a book like this, which discusses natural healthcare, may expect the author to discuss the use of herbs for healing. Indeed, a variety of herbs, such as hawthorn, garlic and mistletoe, are effective in treating various aspects of CVD. However, I am not discussing them in this book because they are not as fundamental as the nutrients outlined above. CVD doesn't happen due to hawthorn deficiency, but it could come about from vitamin C deficiency, for example. Nevertheless, various herbs can be extremely helpful and when a patient doesn't respond to the basic nutritional therapy, I may often recommend herbs in accordance with my assessment of the patient's needs. An herbalist or a healthcare practitioner trained in herbal medicine can make appropriate recommendations for you.

Omega three essential fatty acid – A double edge sword

Both complementary care practitioners and many medical doctors have come to consider omega three polyunsaturated fatty acid important for the prevention and treatment of cardiovascular disease.

As such, my opinion on the requirement for omega three essential fatty acids (PUFA) may surprise many readers. Let me explain.

I discussed extensively the dangers of consuming too much omega six polyunsaturated fatty acid. The structure of omega three polyunsaturated fatty acid closely resembles the structure of omega six polyunsaturated fatty acid. Both lack hydrogen atoms at several locations, a matter that makes them both highly unstable, and a factor in lipid peroxidation. The main difference between the two has to do with the position of the first double bond, i.e., the location where the first pair of hydrogen atoms is missing from the oil's carbon chain. In omega six oil, that happens at the sixth carbon atom from the beginning of the carbon chain; in omega three, that happens at the third carbon on the oil's carbon chain. Omega three polyunsaturated oil is present in very small amounts, in the form of alpha linolenic acid, in plants. Some of the richest sources include flax seeds, chia seeds, walnuts and hemp seeds. In the human body, plant-based omega three alpha linolenic acid is converted to another form, called eicosapentanoic acid (EPA), by the addition of two carbons (the molecule gets longer). EPA omega three oil can be further modified to docosapentanoic acid (DPA) and docosahexanoic acid (DHA). Animal sources of EPA and DHA consist primarily of fish and DPA can also be obtained from marine mammals, such as seals. Unlike omega six oil, omega three oil is perceived as necessary for human health, and there are numerous studies supporting its benefits. These include improvements in blood pressure, heart rate, platelet aggregation (blood thinning effect), levels of blood triglycerides and ensuring healthy arteries. In the body, some omega three oil is converted to eicosanoids, a group of substances that regulate immune functions, including the reduction of inflammation, at least in the short term.

While this all sounds great, its properties as an unstable oil, prone to lipid peroxidation, concern me and so I rarely recommend its use.

Lipid peroxidation leads to a chain reaction of extensive oxidation that results in cell membrane disruption, internal cellular damage, damage of DNA (which can lead to cancer), and overall inflammation. Oxidation of omega three oil can result in the production of toxic substances. The aldehyde HHE (4-hydroxy, 2-hexenal) is implicated in liver and other cellular damage. MDA (malondialdehyde) is implicated in DNA damage and cancer. Lipofuscin is a substance associated with "aging spots" and, more importantly, cellular degeneration and premature aging.[116]

The following quote is from an article by Dr. Ray Peat titled "The Great Fish Oil Experiment":

> "In declaring EPA and DHA to be safe, the FDA neglected to evaluate their anti-thyroid, immunosuppressive, lipid peroxidative (Song et al., 2000), light sensitizing, and anti-mitochondrial effects, their depression of glucose oxidation (Delarue et al., 2003), and

their contribution to metastatic cancer (Klieveri, et al., 2000), lipofuscinosis and liver damage, among other problems".[117]

There is a popular concept that we need to maintain a certain ratio of omega six to omega three oils in our tissues in order to ensure proper health. The consumption of omega six and omega three oils varies widely in various healthy societies around the world, anywhere from 1 part omega three and 4 parts omega six to 4 parts omega three and 1 part omega six[118]. The consumption of omega six PUFA has increased greatly over the course of the twentieth century, to the extent that the ratio has shifted to between 10-20 parts omega six for every one part omega three.

I believe that instead of taking large doses of omega three supplements, we need to focus on reducing the consumption of omega six PUFA in our diet to less than 4% of our daily caloric intake.[119]

The anti-inflammatory effect of omega three oil is not achieved necessarily through tissue repair, but rather by biochemical manipulation of the substances that are involved in immune response. This is similar to the effect of aspirin on inflammation. It is far better and safer to help the body resolve inflammation by limiting the consumption of harmful, inflammation-causing agents, such as omega six PUFA and refined carbohydrates, and by supporting tissue repair (lysine, proline, vitamin C, thyroid support, etc.).

We do need small amounts of the omega three fatty acid metabolite DHA, and, in my opinion, we can get sufficient amounts from food sources such as free-run eggs, fatty fish and grass-fed animals. We can also make it from a plant-based omega three oil, linolenic acid (found in flax seeds, chia seeds, walnuts, etc.).

Based on my understanding of the properties of omega three oil, I don't advocate its long term use as a supplement. Long-term supplementation of omega three oil should be discussed with your healthcare provider first. However, if you or your healthcare provider are convinced of the health benefit of omega three oil supplements, you can take steps to minimize any potential harm (due to tissue oxidation) and optimize their anti-inflammatory benefit by taking them along with some saturated fat (coconut butter or dairy butter, which are far more stable), as well as fat soluble antioxidants, such as vitamins E and A.

Summary Notes

Supplementing with all these nutrients can be overwhelming and you may not need all of them. There are several natural health products on the market that conveniently contain high amount of lysine, proline and vitamin C, along with a number of other key vitamins and minerals, which makes supplementation more convenient and economical. It is best to consult a naturopathic doctor or other qualified natural health practitioner who will assess your health situation and medical history to determine what your specific needs are.

As you implement heart-healthy dietary habits and take the right supplements, you will likely reverse your health condition. Continue monitoring your blood pressure, blood sugar, blood lipids, thyroid hormones and C reactive protein levels. As these factors improve, ask your medical doctor or naturopathic doctor to monitor a gradual reduction in your medications. It has been gratifying to guide many of my clients in decreasing and even eliminating the medications they were on.

CHAPTER 11

MIND-BODY CONNECTION IN CARDIOVASCULAR WELLBEING

Managing Stress

Stress is a factor that influences human health significantly, including cardiovascular wellbeing. A little stress is needed for growth, development and good health, while too much stress is harmful. In this chapter, I will describe what stress is and how it affects human health, especially through its impact on key hormones and on the availability of energy to sustain life. I will also offer some suggestions on ways to reduce unhealthy stress levels.

What is stress, what are stressful factors?

The Miriam Webster dictionary definition of the word *stress* as it relates to human health is "a physical, chemical, or emotional factor that causes bodily or mental tension and may be a factor in disease causation".

Stressful factors are anything that can potentially drain the body of the energy it requires to sustain itself. Stressful factors can be both physical and non-physical. Physical stress factors can include foods such as polyunsaturated fatty acids and overconsumption of baked goods and sugar, infectious agents, toxins, radiation, over work, etc. Non-physical stress factors are psychological or emotional and stem from the way we perceive and react to external events, situations and inputs. It is the result of our perception of how other people and situations affect us. As a result of our interactions or lack of interactions with people, we can become sad, angry, and anxious and so on.

The effect of stress on the body

Our current understanding of the way the body responds to stress is based on the research of Hans Seyle, an endocrinologist who worked at McGill University in Montreal and the University of Montreal in the early part of the 20th century. Dr. Seyles was a pioneer in the area of stress research. He recognized that prolonged exposure to stress had a significant impact on human health and developed the General Adaptation Response theory, which describes the three steps the body takes in response to stress:

Step 1: The Alarm Stage (Shock) - Your first reaction to stress is the recognition of danger and preparation to deal with the threat. During this phase, the main stress hormones cortisol, adrenaline, and noradrenaline, are released to provide instant energy. Your body alarms you with a sudden jolt of hormonal changes that are designed to provide you with enough energy to handle the threat. No living organism can be maintained continuously in the alarm state. If the stress is great enough to be incompatible with life, then death occurs during the alarm reaction.

Step 2: The Resistance Stage - At this stage everything is working as it should – you have a stressful event, your body alarms you with a sudden jolt of hormonal changes, and you are now immediately equipped with enough energy to handle it. Your body here is also trying to conserve its energy to deal with the stressful factor or situation as long as it is present.

Step 3: The Stage of Exhaustion – If the stressful factor remains and you run out of energy to deal with it, exhaustion sets in and many aspects of your health deteriorate (including a reduced ability to heal the arteries and other structures, so chronic inflammation sets in). While the hormones cortisol, adrenaline and noradrenaline provided you with the initial energy you needed to deal with the stressful situation, when their levels are high for too long, they can also cause many harmful effects.

The excess production of the cortisol hormone can cause damage to cells and muscle tissues by breaking down the protein they are made of into the individual amino acids. These amino acids are then converted to make glucose (required for additional energy needs during stress). Stress-related disorders and disease from cortisol include cardiovascular conditions (such as high blood pressure and stroke) as well as gastric ulcers and high blood sugar levels. At this stage, immunity is markedly reduced as well. High cortisol levels also limit the body's ability to produce adequate amounts of the vital thyroid hormones (T4 and T3). These hormones, especially T3 (which is made from T4) govern your ability to produce energy and are important for maintaining healthy cholesterol and blood pressure levels and healthy arteries. Studies show that low thyroid hormone levels are associated with increased risk of heart attack and stroke.

Excessive levels of the hormone adrenaline results in a surge of blood pressure that can damage blood vessels of the heart and brain – a risk factor in heart attack and stroke.

In addition to an increase in the production of cortisol and adrenaline, prolonged stress also causes an increase in other hormones (such as estrogen, prolactin, and serotonin) and a decrease in thyroid hormone. Both of these events can cause problems.

Increased estrogen promotes cell division for growth and water retention, which is great to support a developing fetus, but can also trigger the development of certain cancers. High estrogen also suppresses adequate production of the thyroid hormones.

Increased prolactin is associated with bone loss, hair loss, insulin resistance, inflammation and poor sleep.

Serotonin, a hormone the pharmaceutical industry has promoted as the hormone of well-being is anything but. Most of the serotonin in our bodies is present in the gastrointestinal tract, not in the brain. Serotonin increases adrenaline and cortisol and estrogen (stress hormones) and makes the intestines more permeable to bacterial toxins and anti-nutrients (gluten, etc.).

Stress hormones in high amounts limit the availability of other important hormones that are essential for maintaining optimal health and are protective against CVD. These important hormones include the thyroid hormone (which I already mentioned), as well as progesterone, testosterone and oxytocin. Adequate progesterone and oxytocin provide women with an improved ability to cope with stress and provide a feeling of relaxation and well-being. Testosterone does the same for men. Dealing with stress constructively can help optimize healthy levels of these protective hormones.

Other symptoms related to chronic stress (or the exhaustion stage) include: emotional tension, irritability, anxiety, depression, inability to concentrate, fatigue, twitching, migraine headaches, frequent urination, loss of appetite, weight loss or weight gain, gastrointestinal disturbances, diarrhea or constipation, inflammatory bowel disease, decreased libido, etc.

Correcting hormonal imbalances is really important to ensure overall good health, including a healthy cardiovascular system. This can be done, in part, by improving one's diet and through individualized treatment involving the prescription of certain herbs, vitamins or bio-identical hormones, if need be. However, when the source of stress is not biological, but emotional in nature, or when associated with poor lifestyle choices, other complementary strategies may be helpful.

The next part of this chapter offers a brief discussion of several approaches to reducing excessive stress and its harmful effect on your health.

Methods and techniques to reduce stress and the impact of stress

Various lifestyle strategies exist to help cope with stress. These include: psychotherapy, following a spiritual practice, practicing meditation, deep breathing exercises, yoga, tai chi or qi gong, exercise, going for walks, as well as other leisure activities such as reading for fun, pursuing a hobby, etc.

I believe that psychotherapy and engaging in spiritual teachings and practices are the most important strategies for dealing with chronic stress. These methods help people re-evaluate their beliefs and values in order to make the necessary changes (internal and external) to reach a greater sense of fulfillment and peace of mind.

For example, I had a patient who had hypertension due to stress from an abusive relationship. She chose to seek counselling, while her partner refused counselling and didn't stop the abuse. Through this process she summoned the courage and the self-esteem she needed to end the relationship. Shortly after, her blood pressure improved dramatically. In this case, this woman had to make some internal changes to her way of thinking and increase her sense of self-worth in order to take the steps that helped her body heal.

Another patient with hypertension was very critical of her daughter and son-in-law and was resentful towards them. As an objective observer, I saw that she chose to see herself as the victim in this relationship. After ruling out and addressing all the biological causes of her hypertension, it became clear to me that her constant state of anger was keeping her blood pressure up. I recommended that she seek counselling, but she refused. I was unable to help her deal with the source of stress in her life that caused her hypertension.

Another common example is overwork, sometimes driven by a need to earn enough money to survive, but sometimes driven by a false sense of lack of self-worth, the belief that "my worth depends on how financially successful I am, and so I need to work continuously, until I reach enough financial success to prove my worthiness". No matter what the reason is, overwork can lead to poor physical health, or to unhealthy family relationships, lack of peace of mind and lack of true happiness.

Often, a change in our belief system, in our perspective on life, re-prioritizing what is important and what isn't, can bring a greater sense of balance to life and help turn our health around.

Physical activity

Regular exercise has been shown to be as effective as drug therapy for mild to moderate depression and anxiety and as means to reduce stress.

In terms of cardiovascular risk factors, regular physical exercise has many benefits:

- Increase in exercise tolerance
- Reduction in body weight
- Reduction in blood pressure
- Reduction in LDL and total cholesterol
- Increase in HDL cholesterol
- Increase in insulin sensitivity (decreased resistance)
- Increase in life expectancy

According to a paper published by Jonathan Myers, PhD in the medical journal *Circulation*, several public health and medical agencies (The Surgeon General's Report, a joint CDC/ACSM consensus statement, and a National Institutes of Health report) all agreed that the benefits I listed above will generally occur by engaging in at least thirty minutes of modest activity on most, preferably all, days of the week.

"Modest activity is defined as any activity that is similar in intensity to brisk walking at a rate of about three to four miles per hour. These activities include any other form of occupational or recreational activity that is dynamic in nature and of similar intensity, such as cycling, yard work, and swimming". [120] The thirty minutes spent being physically active is cumulative; it doesn't need to be done all at once.

A great type of physical activity that can both improve your fitness level and help you relax is yoga. Through stretching and focus on deep breathing, yoga helps deliver more oxygen to tissues, lower the production of stress hormones, increase the production of oxytocin (a relaxation hormone), and so increase feelings of relaxation and wellbeing. A systemic review of seventy studies concluded that yoga may reduce many risk factors related to CVD. [121] Tai Chi, a type of Chinese martial art practiced for both its defense training and its health benefits, has also been shown to be beneficial for improving cardiovascular well-being. [122]

If you find it challenging to start exercising on a regular basis, start by making simple choices and engage in activities you enjoy. Something is absolutely better than nothing. Here are some examples, in no particular order: Climb stairs instead of taking the elevator, park at the end of a parking lot, have a "walk-meeting", invite someone for a walk, get a dog that you need to walk, walk to the store, engage in gardening and yard activities, join a fitness class, ride a stationary bike in front of the TV, replace coffee breaks with walking breaks, go skating or tobogganing with the kids or grandkids, play football or baseball with them, etc.

Kicking Harmful Habits

Regular use of cigarettes and alcohol are habits some people may form to try to cope with stress and to relax. It is well known that both of these habits have harmful effects on the cardiovascular system.

Women who drink more than one alcoholic drink a day and men who drink more than two alcoholic beverages are at a greater risk of developing arrhythmia, hypertension, hemorrhagic (bleeding) stroke, fatty liver, insulin resistance and more.[123]

Nicotine, carbon monoxide and other toxins in cigarettes are substances that cause oxidation. These substances damage the lining of the arteries through oxidation, leading to the development of atherosclerosis, increasing the risk of a heart attack and stroke.

The addiction to these or any other harmful substances (drugs) or harmful habits (gambling, over-eating) stem from a constant underlying need to fill a void or a lack, often a subconscious lack in life. It could be a lack of happiness, a perceived lack of love, approval, self-worth, guilt, and a general lack of fulfillment. Often talk therapy, psychotherapy, group therapy and hypnotherapy can help uncover these causes and help bring awareness of the underlying cause for the addictions. These strategies may or may not resolve the addictions right away; ultimately, it is up to each and every person to summon the will to resolve harmful habits. The widely-popular Alcoholics Anonymous organization, for example, has been successful at helping many people "kick the habit" through their group therapy support system. It provides a safe environment to allow participants to discover and address the underlying causes of their alcohol addiction.

There are additional strategies to help people resolve these types of unhealthy habits. Naturopathic doctors and natural health practitioners use herbal preparations, nutrition and acupuncture to help improve the ability to cope with stress and to diminish cravings for nicotine or alcohol. Recently, I have become aware of laser acupuncture therapy as a means to help reduce cravings. A laser therapy practitioner showed me how he applies a probe with a pointer emitting laser waves at specific acupuncture points on the ear, which helps lessen the craving to smoke.

Healthy lifestyle choices go hand in hand with healthy nutrition to help ensure a strong and healthy cardiovascular system. In fact, a study published in *The Lancet* showed that dietary and lifestyle intervention alone can help reverse coronary heart disease without the use of drugs.[124]

CHAPTER 12

HOW DO YOU KNOW IF YOUR PIPES ARE CLOGGED UP?

Different Ways to Assess Risk

There are blood tests and imaging procedures that are helpful at discerning whether you have some measure of atherosclerosis or outright blockages in the arteries. However, before you even go to get tested, what signs and symptoms should you look out for? There are certain signs that could indicate atherosclerosis or the existence of plaque in the arteries.

Signs to watch out for

- *Hypertension*: As discussed, the vast majority of high blood pressure cases are associated with narrowing of the arteries.

- *Pulse Pressure*: This helps to interpret your blood pressure reading in a way that more accurately predicts whether you have atherosclerosis and plaque build-up. Pulse pressure refers to the difference between the upper reading (systolic) of your blood pressure and bottom (diastolic) reading of your blood pressure. So, for example, the way you calculate the pulse pressure of a healthy blood pressure reading of 120/80 is by subtraction: 120-80=40. The pulse pressure here is 40. A pulse pressure higher than 40 is not considered normal and may have various causes, such as acute hyperthyroidism, aortic regurgitation, fever, anemia, endocarditis, and so on. However, when those conditions aren't present and when both the blood pressure and the pulse pressure are high, especially as the pulse pressure creeps past 50, it is a likely sign of the presence of atherosclerosis. Don't confuse the term "pulse pressure" with the tern "pulse", which simply refers to the heart rate.

- *Shortness of breath* with no physical activity or relatively slight exertion, such as climbing up a flight of stairs or going for a brisk walk.

- *Constantly cold hands and feet* (regardless of the environment's temperature) may be an indication of poor circulation due to narrowed arteries.

- *The presence of uncontrolled diabetes* is a sure sign that plaque is being formed. Unfortunately, many people with diabetes think that it is controlled when blood sugar levels drop to eight or seven; however, controlled blood sugar levels are levels that are considered normal for healthy, non-diabetic people.

- Most importantly, everyone should be familiar with *signs of a heart attack*, which include: chest pain, chest discomfort (uncomfortable chest pressure, squeezing, fullness or pain, burning or heaviness), discomfort in other areas of the upper body (neck, jaw, shoulder, arms, back), shortness of breath, profuse sweating, debilitating, flulike exhaustion, light headedness, nausea and/or dizziness.

Blood tests

Since high total cholesterol isn't a good indication of your risk for cardiovascular disease, what other measures can you rely on? There are some other substances you can be tested for that offer a good indication of your risk level. It is important that you always ask for a copy of your test results, so you can track changes each time you get a blood test. By law, your healthcare providers are obliged to provide you with a copy. Expect to pay a nominal administrative fee if you request a copy of your entire file.

C reactive protein (CRP)

Studies show that measuring inflammation is one good way of determining your risk. One of the substances in the blood that more and more doctors are looking for is C reactive protein or CRP. CRP levels rise with inflammation. Because atherosclerosis, the laying down of plaque, is driven by inflammation, high CRP levels are associated with greater risk.

However, CRP can be high due to inflammation that is associated with other health issues, such as arthritis, inflammatory skin disease or recent injuries. Because the dietary causes of arthritis are often the same as the dietary causes of cardiovascular disease, both conditions generally go hand in hand. However, if you had a recent injury, inflammation set in to heal the injured area and your CRP will likely be high; therefore, in a case of recent injury, CRP is not a valuable indicator to assess your risk of cardiovascular disease. Other factors and blood test markers need to be considered.

High density lipo-protein (HDL)

If your good cholesterol is too low, you may potentially be in trouble. As mentioned earlier, HDL carries cholesterol back from the blood into the cells of the liver, the adrenal glands, ovaries and testes. Therefore, doctors who still follow the notion that cholesterol is the cause of atherosclerosis see the HDL benefit as a cholesterol-removing agent. However, in addition to this role of HDL, it also helps

123

to inhibit oxidation, inflammation and coagulation (stickiness of the blood), all processes that contribute to atherosclerosis. Therefore, low levels of HDL constitute a prime risk factor for atherosclerosis.

Triglycerides

These are fat storage molecules. In high amounts, they increase the risk for cardiovascular disease. Presence of high triglycerides is correlated with excessive intake of refined carbohydrates. One study showed that high carbohydrate intake (60% of the total daily caloric intake) increases blood levels of triglycerides.[125]

Fasting insulin

This is something doctors usually don't test for, but they easily could. I discussed the relationship between insulin and sugar and CVD. Indeed, several studies have confirmed this relationship.[126, 127, 128, 129] Elevated blood levels of insulin is an indication that cells don't respond to insulin very well, and so it doesn't function efficiently at driving glucose into the cells. Glucose that lingers in the blood stream causes glycation (stickiness) of the arteries.

Lipo-protein A (Lp(a))

Lp(a) is derived from cholesterol; however, its risk factor has nothing to do with the amount of cholesterol in your blood. Dr. Pauling and Dr. Rath considered it to be an important risk factor. Their research showed that the amount of Lp(a) in plaque in coronary arteries and certain arteries that feed the brain is far greater than the amount of cholesterol.

They suggested that Lp(a) acts as a "band aid", sticking to areas of damaged arteries in an attempt to repair them.[130] When Lp(a) sticks to the arteries, it contributes directly to atherosclerosis. The amount of Lp(a) can vary a thousand times from one person to another. It varies greatly among races (people of African descent have the highest amount) and genetics plays a role here, more than with any other blood risk factor. People who have normal CRP, HDL and triglyceride levels who have been diagnosed with CVD, or had a heart attack or a stroke, should consider getting tested for Lp(a).

Thyroid hormones (TSH, T4, T3)
Research shows that people with an underactive thyroid (hypothyroidism) are more prone to develop plaque in the arteries. [131] Sometimes a thyroid function test may come back as "normal", but if symptoms of hypothyroidism exist, hypothyroidism needs to be considered because it is an important risk factor. Refer to the section on the mineral iodine in Chapter Ten to recall what the symptoms of hypothyroidism are.

Fibrinogen
Fibrinogen is a protein in your blood that helps blood clot. But too much fibrinogen can cause a clot to form in an artery, leading to a heart attack or stroke. Having too much fibrinogen may also mean that you have atherosclerosis. It may also worsen existing injury to artery walls.

125

Other substances

There are other substances in the blood that can offer insight into your risk for cardiovascular disease (such as homocysteine or apolipoprotein B). However, I won't discuss them here since blood tests for these factors are more uncommon and you have got enough to work with using the other factors listed in this chapter.

Kidney function markers

Poor kidney function can, among other reasons, be the result of long term use of certain heart meds. It can also result from long standing hypertension or, conversely, contribute to hypertension. Assessing kidney function may often be required for proper treatment. Early signs of poor kidney function include protein or blood in the urine and a high albumin to creatinine ratio. More progressive poor kidney function is diagnosed by low eGFR (glomerular filtration rate) and the gold standard, high creatinine levels.

Imaging Tests

Coronary angiogram

A coronary angiogram is a procedure that uses X-ray imaging to see your heart's blood vessels. Coronary angiograms are part of a general group of procedures known as cardiac catheterization.

Heart catheterization procedures can both diagnose and treat heart and blood vessel conditions. A coronary angiogram, which can help diagnose heart conditions, is the most common type of heart catheter procedure.

During a coronary angiogram, a type of dye that's visible by X-ray machine is injected into the blood vessels of your heart. The X-ray machine rapidly takes a series of images (angiograms) offering a detailed look at the inside of your blood vessels.

If necessary, your doctor can perform procedures such as angioplasty during your coronary angiogram. This is usually done for people who already have evidence of blockages, such as chest pain and symptoms of a heart attack, and for those with cardiac valve disease. It is not offered to anyone who has no other evidence of arterial blockages.

CT coronary angiogram

A computerized tomography (CT) coronary angiogram is an imaging test to look at the arteries that supply your heart muscle with blood. Unlike a traditional coronary angiogram, CT angiograms don't use a catheter threaded through your blood vessels to your heart. Instead, a coronary CT angiogram relies on a powerful X-ray machine to produce images of your heart and heart vessels. CT angiograms will expose you to a small amount of radiation.

Coronary CT angiograms are becoming a common option for people with a variety of heart conditions. This is suitable for individuals who don't have symptoms yet, but based on age and other factors (such as high blood pressure and smoking) may be at greater risk.

Coronary calcium scans

Heart scans, also known as coronary calcium scans, provide pictures of your heart's arteries (coronary arteries). Doctors use heart scans to look for calcium deposits in the coronary arteries. Calcium deposits can narrow your arteries and increase your heart attack risk. The result of this test is often called a coronary calcium score.

Heart scans may show that you have a higher risk of having a heart attack or other problems before you have any obvious symptoms of heart disease. Like the CT, this too is best suited for people with moderate risk. However, this type of test is rarely administered and is generally offered through private clinics.

Carotid artery ultrasound

The carotid arteries (one on each side of the neck) supply blood to the rest of the brain. An ultrasound of these two arteries is a non-invasive technique used to detect plaque in these arteries and to predict the risk of developing a stroke (due to blockage in the arteries of the brain). Studies show that plaque developed on the carotid arteries is also predictive of plaque developed elsewhere in the body, including the coronary arteries of the heart.[132]

Unlike an angiogram, an ultrasound image is not as precise and it shows plaque accumulation in 25% increments. However, because this test is safe, easy and inexpensive, it is a viable tool to help assess risk.

In-Office Tests

Ankle-brachial index

The ankle-brachial index test is a quick, noninvasive, in-office way to check your risk of peripheral artery disease (PAD). Peripheral artery disease is a condition in which the arteries in your legs or arms are narrowed or blocked. The ankle-brachial index test compares your blood pressure measured at your ankle with your blood pressure measured at your arm. A low ankle-brachial index number can indicate narrowing or blockage of the arteries in your legs, leading to circulatory problems, heart disease or stroke. People with peripheral artery disease are at a high risk of heart attack, stroke, poor circulation and leg pain.

Becoming familiar with these signs and tests will hopefully allow you to better gauge your risk level and will enable you to engage in a meaningful dialogue with your doctor when need be.

129

CHAPTER 13

WHO'S ON YOUR TEAM AND WHAT POSITION DO THEY PLAY?

Try Integrating the Best of Both Worlds

Bridging the gap between conventional and natural healthcare

There is a gap to be bridged between the allopathic (currently conventional) medical model and natural healthcare. Currently, doctors get very little training in nutrition. They are also obliged by their regulatory bodies to follow pharmaceutical-based protocols. Their information comes from studies presented by pharmaceutical reps, and medical conferences and medical journals which are sponsored by pharmaceutical companies, and much of the information is driven by their agenda.

Most practitioners, including myself, are too busy to spend time reading studies in their entirety and analyzing their value and objectivity. Only a small portion of doctors choose to get training in nutritional and natural therapies and use them to treat patients.

In my experience, most doctors would not express opposition to your nutritional program as long as it is working and as long as they feel that you are doing it safely. Some may raise objections. A doctor's objection to a natural treatment may be the reason why some people choose not to inform their doctor of the nutritional supplements they are taking or the natural therapies they are engaged in. However, your medical doctor plays an important part in healthcare delivery and you should inform him or her of whatever complementary approaches you use to improve your health, regardless of any possible objection on their part. Ask your doctor to monitor changes in your condition and help adjust your meds accordingly. Most doctors wouldn't be averse to doing this.

Your pharmacist can also play an important role. In my experience, most pharmacists, are far more concerned about poly-pharmacy (the use of multiple medications simultaneously), than medical doctors, who often simply follow prescription protocols. A pharmacist can review your list of medications and, if need be, mediate discussions about any possible safety or efficacy concerns.

If your doctor resists your wish to try the approach presented in this book, you have a decision to make.

Ultimately, it is your body and it is your responsibility to educate yourself and decide what is best for your health.

Having said that, a recent randomized control study published in a mainstream medical journal confirmed the benefits of naturopathic treatment for the management of cardiovascular disease. The premise of the study was the idea that "Although cardiovascular disease may be partially preventable through dietary and lifestyle-based interventions, few individuals at risk receive intensive dietary and lifestyle counselling."[133] This book certainly offers "intensive dietary and life style counselling". However, what it cannot offer is an individualized treatment plan. The medium for an individualized treatment plan is an in-office consult with a naturopathic doctor, a medical doctor trained in natural medicine or with other licensed practitioners in your jurisdiction who are trained in modalities of natural medicine.

An individualized treatment plan offers several important benefits. In this book, I tried to help you learn how to deal with the general, common causes of CVD (glycation, oxidation and inflammation), brought about by dietary and lifestyle factors. However, everybody is different, and different people may require different types of treatments or intervention. Factors that may influence your ability to get better include, person-specific hormonal imbalance, kidney disease, autoimmune disease, digestive concerns, allergies, etc. A naturopathic doctor can requisition relevant tests and guide you accordingly.

A naturopathic doctor can provide you with the comfort level and the self-assurance you need to make the transition from a medicated to a non-medicated approach (to the extent that it is possible, since sometimes, some medications may be required).

Also, your naturopathic doctor can communicate with your MD in "medical language" about your treatment plan and about any concerns that need to be addressed. Ideally, you would integrate the best of both worlds, the conventional medical model and the natural medical model.

A brief note about the qualifications of naturopathic doctors

Make sure to work with a naturopathic doctor (ND) who is licensed or – in unlicensed jurisdictions – someone who was schooled in a legitimate, accredited naturopathic medical school. Go to the web site of the Council on Naturopathic Medical Education at *www.cnme.org* to find a list of accredited schools.

Naturopathic medical schooling consists of four years of full-time intensive studies after having completed an undergraduate degree. It involves the study of both basic medical sciences (anatomy, pathology, etc.) and natural treatment modalities (herbs, nutrition, acupuncture and homeopathy).

The word doctor means "teacher" in Latin. The primary role of a naturopathic doctor is to teach clients how to care for their own health. You can imagine that if I had to teach all the information I provided you in this book in my office, you would have to come in for many office visits. Of course, information merely gives you a chance, the potential to turn around your health. Information needs to be turned into practice. It has to be acted on, and for this additional guidance may be required.

Because of the importance of the information this book delivers and because there is a need to turn this information into action, I launched a special multi-class program designed to further educate, inform and guide you towards markedly improved health. It is called *Dr. Klein's Revolutionary Healthy Heart Program™*.

You can view the first class of the program at *www.drkleinhealthyheart.com*.

Many of those who follow my program experience significant improvements in their health (blood pressure, cholesterol, blood sugar etc.).

I wish that you enjoy great health as you move forward to implement what you learned in this book.

Appendix

Additional Resources Available on:
www.DrKleinHealthyHeart.com

On my website I provide you with links to additional resources to help you on your journey to better health.

Personal Resources

- My personal blog with continuously added articles and new findings on health and wellness

- My free video of class number one of Dr. Klein's Healthy Heart Program™

The truth about cholesterol, blood pressure and fat

- The International Network of Cholesterol Skeptics (*www.thincs.org/links.htm*): a long list of articles by many researchers

- "LDL Cholesterol: 'Bad' Cholesterol or bad science" (*http://www.thincs.org/links.htm*): A brilliant review of the cholesterol folly published in the *Journal of American Physicians and Surgeons*

- *The Cholesterol Myths* by Dr. Uffe Ravnskov (*http://www.ravnskov.nu/cholesterol.htm#*) A free book with mountains of references about the truth on cholesterol

- The Weston A. Price Foundation (*http://www.westonaprice.org/*): The website of the Weston A. Price foundation, an excellent resource on nutrition

Favorite Researchers

- *www.raypeat.com*: Ray Peat, Ph.D., offers not so politically correct, scientifically backed articles on health (not an easy read without a background in science)

- *http://wholehealthsource.blogspot.ca*: Stephan Guyenet, Ph.D., writes a blog that focuses on the science of obesity and related matters

- *www.mercola.com*: Doctor Mercola has done a great job at debunking common myths about health and disease, and promoting natural approaches to well-being

Resources on Food and Nutrition

- *www.data.self.com*: Nutrition facts, including food labels, calories, nutritional information and analysis that helps promote healthy eating by telling you about the foods you eat.

- *www.whfoods.com:* Non-profit foundation providing reliable, scientifically accurate, personalized information for convenient and enjoyable healthy eating

Resources on Pharmaceutical Medications

- *www.drugs.com*
- *www.rxlist.com*

Health Library

- *http://www.umm.edu/altmed*: The online health library of the University of Maryland Medical Centre

[1] Eileen T et al. "Dietary fat Intake in the US Population". *JACN*, vol 18, no3

[2] Sodium Intake Estimates for 2003–2006 and Description of Dietary Sources, *NCBI*, http://www.ncbi.nlm.nih.gov/books/NBK50960/ accessed 01/20/2013

[3] Heart Disease and Stroke Statistics–2006 Update. *Circulation.* 2006;113:e85-e151

[4] Heart Disease and Stroke Statistics—2012 Update. *Circulation.* 2012; 125: e2-e220

[5] Zhang Q, Wang Y, Huang ES. "Changes in racial/ethnic disparities in the prevalence of Type 2 diabetes by obesity level among US adults". *Ethn Health.* 2009;14:439–457

[6] Fast Stats, Leading Causes of Death. Centers for Disease Control and Prevention. http://www.cdc.gov/nchs/fastats/lcod.html Date of retrieval June 24, 2013

[7] Statistics. Heart and Stroke Foundation. http://www.heartandstroke.com/site/c.iklQLcMWJtE/b.3483991/. Date of retrieval June 24, 2013

[8] Media Centre, Cardiovascular Disease. World Health Organization. Updated March 2013. http://www.who.int/mediacentre/factsheets/fs317/en/, retrieved June 24, 2013

[9] Heart Disease and Stroke Statistics–2006 Update. *Circulation.* 2006;113:e85-e151

[10] Heart Disease and Stroke Statistics—2012 Update. *Circulation.* 2012; 125: e2-e220

[11] Statehealthfacts.org, Retail Prescription Drugs Filled at Pharmacies (Annual per Capita by Age), 2010

[12] Diao D, Wright JM, Cundiff DK, Gueyffier F. "Pharmacotherapy for mild hypertension". *Cochrane Database of Systematic Reviews* 2012, Issue 8. Art. No.: CD006742. DOI:10.1002/14651858.CD006742.pub2

[13] Sripal Bangalore, "β-Blocker Use and Clinical Outcomes in Stable Outpatients With and Without Coronary Artery Disease". *JAMA.* 2012;308(13):1340-1349. doi:10.1001/jama.2012.12559

[14] Bangalore, S., *et al.* "A meta-analysis of 94,492 patients with hypertension treated with beta blockers to determine the risk of new-onset diabetes mellitus". *Am J. Cardiol.* 2007 Oct 15;100(8):1254-62.

[15] Lindholm LH, Carlberg B, Samuelsson O. "Should beta blockers remain first choice in the treatment of primary hypertension? A meta-analysis". *Lancet.* 2005;366:1545–53.

[16] Psaty BM, Heckbert SR, Koepsell TD, Siscovick DS, et al. "The risk of myocardial infarction associated with antihypertensive drug therapies". *JAMA* 1995;274:620-5.

[17] Eisenberg MJ, Brox A, Bestawros AN. "Calcium channel blockers: an update". *Am J Med* 2004; 116:35.

[18] Alan J. Zillich et al. "Thiazide Diuretics, Potassium, and the Development of Diabetes". *Hypertension. 2006;48:219-224*

[19] Graham J. Frank. "The Safety of ACE Inhibitors for the Treatment of Hypertension and Congestive Heart Failure". *Kidney International* 2006; 69: 913–919

[20] Angiotensin II receptor agonists, Wkipidia, http://en.wikipedia.org/wiki/Angiotensin_II_receptor_antagonist#cite_note-Rossi-9. Date of retrieval an 12 2013

[21] Strauss MH, Hall AS (2006). "Angiotensin receptor blockers may increase risk of myocardial infarction: unraveling the ARB-MI paradox". *Circulation* 114 (8): 838–54

[22] Naveed Sattar PhD et al., "Statins and risk of incident diabetes: a collaborative meta-analysis of randomised statin trials". *The Lancet,* Volume 375, Issue 9716, Pages 735 - 742, 27 February 2010

[23] *Andrew Mente, PhD; Lawrence de Koning, MSc; Harry S. Shannon, PhD; Sonia S. Anand, MD, PhD, FRCPC,* "A Systematic Review of the Evidence Supporting a Causal Link Between Dietary Factors and Coronary Heart Disease". *Arch Intern Med.* 2009; 169(7):659-669

[24] Newman TB, Hulley SB, "Carcinogenicity of lipid-lowering drugs". *JAMA.* 1996 Jan 3;275(1):55-60

[25] Sachdeva A, Cannon CP, Deedwania PC, Labresh KA, Smith SC Jr, Dai D, Hernandez A, Fonarow GC., "Lipid levels in patients hospitalized with coronary artery disease: an analysis of 136,905 hospitalizations in Get With The Guidelines". *Am Heart J.* 2009 Jan; 157(1):111-117.

[26] Al-Mallah MH et al. "Low admission LDL-cholesterol is associated with increased 3-year all-cause mortality in patients with non ST segment elevation myocardial infarction". *Cardiol J.* 2009;16(3):227-33.

[27] Kastelein JJ et al. "Simvastatin with or without ezetimibe in familial hypercholesterolemia". *N Engl J Med.* 2008 Apr 3; 358(14):1431-43.

[28] AWE Weverling-Rijnsburger, et al. "Total cholesterol and risk of mortality in the oldest old". *Lancet* 1997; 350: 1119-23.

[29] Meilahn, Elaine M., "Low serum Cholesterol Hazardous to Your Health?", *Circulation.* 1995; 92: 2365-2366

[30] Sarria Cabrera MA, et al. " Lipids and all-cause mortality among older adults: a 12-year follow-up study". *Scientific World Journal Epub* 1 May 2012

[31] Keaven M. Anderson, PhD; William P. Castelli, MD; Daniel Levy, MD. "Cholesterol and Mortality 30 Years of Follow-up From the Framingham Study". *JAMA* 1987;257:2176-2180

[32] Naila rabani Et al. "Glycation of LDL by Methylglyoxal Increases Arterial Atherogenicity. A Possible Contributor to Increased Risk of Cardiovascular Disease in Diabetes". *Diabetes* May 2011

[33] Mary Enig Ph.D., The Skinny on Fat, http://www.westonaprice.org/know-your-fats/skinny-on-fats, Jun 2012, published Jan 2000

[34] Stephan Guyenet. The coronary Heart DieaseEpidemic: Possible Culprits Part 2. Whole Health Source, Tuesday may 19 2009. http://wholehealthsource.blogspot.ca/2009/05/coronary-heart-disease-epidemic_19.html; Date of Retrieval: Feb 13 2013

[35] Mary G. Enig, PhD and Sally Fallon. "The oiling of America". The Weston A. Price Foundation. http://www.westonprice.org/know-your-fats/the-oiling-of-america. (August 2 2011).

[36] Heini AF, Weinsier RL. "Divergent trends in obesity and fat intake patterns: the American paradox". *Am J Med*. 1997 Mar;102(3):259-64

[37] Hodan Farah Wells, Jean C. Buzby. Dietary Assessment of Consumption, 1970-2005, USDA, March 2008, economic information bulletin #33, http://www.ers.usda.gov/publications/eib33/eib33.pdf (June 2012)

[38] Eileen T. Kennedy et al. "Dietary fat intake in the US population". *Journal of the American College of Nutrition*, Vol. 18, No. 3, 207–212 (1999)

[39] Mente A, et al. "A systematic review of the evidence supporting a causal link between dietary factors and coronary heart disease". *Arch Intern Med*. 2009 Apr 13;169(7):659-69

[40] Siri-Tarino PW, et al. "Meta-analysis of prospective cohort studies evaluating the association of saturated fat with cardiovascular disease". *Am J Clin Nutr*. 2010 Mar;91(3):535-46.

[41] Hooper L, et al. "Reduced or modified dietary fat for preventing cardiovascular disease". Cochrane Database Syst Rev. 2011 Jul 6;(7):CD002137.

[42] *Nourishing Traditions: The Cookbook that Challenges Politically Correct Nutrition and the Diet Dictocrats* by Sally Fallon with Mary G. Enig, PhD (NewTrends Publishing 2000, www.newtrendspublishing.com 877-707-1776)

[43] Andrew Mente, PhD; Lawrence de Koning, MSc; Harry S. Shannon, PhD; Sonia S. Anand, MD, PhD, FRCPC, "A Systematic Review of the Evidence Supporting a Causal Link Between Dietary Factors and Coronary Heart Disease". *Arch Intern Med*. 2009; 169(7):659-669

[44] Geoffrey Rose et al. "Intersalt". *BMJ*. 1988 July 30; 297(6644): 319–328.

[45] Intersalt Cooperative Research Group. "Intersalt: an international study of electrolyte excretion and blood pressure. Results for 24

hour urinary sodium and potassium excretion". *BMJ*. 1988;297(6644):319-328

[46] Miller JZ, Weinberger MH, Daugherty SA, Fineberg, NS, Christian JC, Grim CE. "Heterogeneity of blood pressure response to dietary sodium restriction in normotensive adults". *J Chron Dis*. 1987:40(3):245-250.

[47] Alderman et al. "Association of Renin-Sodium Profile with the Risk of Myocardial Infarction in Patients with Hypertension", 324 *N. Engl. J. Med*. 1098-1104 (1991).

[48] Alderman MH, Cohen H, Madhavan S. "Dietary sodium intake and mortality: the National Health and Nutrition Examination Survey (NHANES I)". *Lancet*. 1998;351(9105):781-5

[49] Cohen HW, Hailpern SM, Fang J, Alderman MH, "Sodium intake and mortality in the NHANES II follow-up study". *Am J Med*. 2006;119(3):275.e7-14.

[50] Cohen HW, Hailpern SM, Alderman MH, "Sodium intake and mortality follow-up in the Third National Health and Nutrition Examination Survey (NHANES III)". *J Gen Intern Med*. 2008;23(9):1297-302.

[51] Graudal NA, Hubeck-Graudal T, Jürgens G. "Effects of low-sodium diet vs. high-sodium diet on blood pressure, renin, aldosterone, catecholamines, cholesterol, and triglyceride (Cochrane Review)". *Am J Hypertens* 2011;25:1–15.

[52] Nakandakare et al. "Dietary salt restriction increases plasma lipoprotein and inflammatory marker concentrations in hypertensive patients". *Atherosclerosis* 200(2): 410-16 (2008).

[53] Andrew Mente, PhD; Lawrence de Koning, MSc; Harry S. Shannon, PhD; Sonia S. Anand, MD, PhD, FRCPC, "A Systematic Review of the Evidence Supporting a Causal Link Between Dietary Factors and Coronary Heart Disease". *Arch Intern Med*. 2009; 169(7):659-669

[54] Wahjudi et al, "Carbohydrate Analysis of High Fructose Corn Syrup (HFCS) Containing Commercial Beverages". *The Faseb Journal*, Apr 2010

[55] Ki-Bum Won, MD et al. "High serum advanced glycation end-products predict coronary artery disease irrespective of arterial

stiffness in diabetic patients". *Korean Circ J.* 2012 May; 42(5): 335–340

[56] Peppa M et al. "Advanced glycation end products and cardiovascular disease". *Curr Diabetes Rev.* 2008 May;4(2):92-100.

[57] Simm A, Wagner J, Gursinsky T, Nass N, Friedrich I, Schinzel R, Czeslik E, Silber RE, Scheubel RJ. "Advanced glycation endproducts: a biomarker for age as an outcome predictor after cardiac surgery?" *Exp Gerontol.* 2007 Jul;42(7):668-75.

[58] Williams S. Harris et al. AHA Science Advisory, "Omega-6 Fatty Acids and Risk for Cardiovascular Disease". *Circulation.* 2009; 119: 902-907

[59] Mozaffarian D, Micha R, Wallace S (2010) "Effects on Coronary Heart Disease of Increasing Polyunsaturated Fat in Place of Saturated Fat: A Systematic Review and Meta-Analysis of Randomized Controlled Trials". *PLoS Med* 7(3)

[60] Diet-Heart Controlled Trials: a New Literature Review, Stephan Guyenet, Whole Health Source.
http://wholehealthsource.blogspot.ca/2010/12/diet-heart-controlled-trials-new.html Dec 2 2010. Date of retrieval Jan 13, 2013

[61] Christopher E. Ramsden." n-6 Fatty acid-specific and mixed polyunsaturate dietary interventions have different effects on CHD risk: a meta-analysis of randomised controlled trials". *British Journal of Nutrition* (2010), 104, 1586–1600.
doi:10.1017/S0007114510004010

[62] Felton, CV, et al, *Lancet,* 1994, 344:1195

[63] Stephan Guynet. Eicosanoids and Ischemic Heart Disease, Part II. Whole health Source. May 27 2009. Date of retrieval Dec 31 2012. http://wholehealthsource.blogspot.ca/2009/05/eicosanoids-and-ischemic-heart-diseas.html#uds-search-results

[64] Lands WE, "Biochemistry and physiology of n-3 fatty acids". *FASEB J.* 1992 May;6(8):2530-6.

[65] J. Girard, "Role of free fatty acids in insulin resistance of subjects with non-insulin-dependent diabetes," *Diabetes Metab.* 21(2), 79-88,1995

[66] Halade GV. "High fat diet-induced animal model of age-associated obesity and osteoporosis". *J Nutr Biochem*. 2010 Dec;21(12):1162-9

[67] Henriksen T, Mahoney EM, Steinberg D. "Enhanced macrophage degradation of biologically modified low density lipoprotein". *Arteriosclerosis*. Mar-Apr 1983;3(2):149-159

[68] Nagy L, Tontonoz P, Alvarez JG, Chen H, Evans RM. "Oxidized LDL regulates macrophage gene expression through ligand activation of PPARgamma". *Cell*. Apr 17 1998;93(2):229-240

[69] DM van Reyk and W Jessup. "The macrophage in atherosclerosis: modulation of cell function by sterols". *Journal of Leukocyte Biology*, Vol 66, Issue 4 557-561

[70] Mireille Ouimet et al. "Epoxycholesterol Impairs Cholesteryl Ester Hydrolysis in Macrophage Foam Cells, Resulting in Decreased Cholesterol Efflux". *Arteriosclerosis, Thrombosis, and Vascular Biology*. 2008;28:1144-1150

[71] Fu MX, Requena JR, Jenkins AJ, Lyons TJ, Baynes JW, Thorpe SR. Nepsilon. "The advanced glycation end product, Nepsilon-(carboxymethyl) lysine, is a product of both lipid peroxidation and glycoxidation reactions". *J Biol Chem* 1996 Apr 26;271(17):9982-6.

[72] Andrew Mente, PhD; Lawrence de Koning, MSc; Harry S. Shannon, PhD; Sonia S. Anand, MD, PhD, FRCPC, "A Systematic Review of the Evidence Supporting a Causal Link Between Dietary Factors and Coronary Heart Disease". *Arch Intern Med*. 2009; 169(7):659-669

[73] Fred A. Kummerow, "The negative effects of hydrogenated trans fats and what to do about them". *Atherosclerosis*; Aug 2009; Volume 205, Issue 2: 458-465

[74] Trelle, S., Reichenbach, S., Wandel, S, et al. "Cardiovascular safety of non-steroidal anti-inflammatory drugs: network meta-analysis". *BMJ* 2011; 342

[75] Pribilia et al. Improved Lactose Digestion and Intolerance Among African-American Adolescent Girls Fed a Dairy Rich-Diet Journal of the American Dietetic Association; **Volume 100, Issue 5**, Pages 524-528, May 2000

[76] Frederic W. Douglas Jr. Et al. "Effects of ultra-high-temperature pasteurization on milk proteins". *J. Agric. Food Chem.*, 1981, 29 (1), pp 11–15. DOI: 10.1021/jf00103a004

[77] Long, C. and Newbury, U. "The Good Egg." *Mother Earth News,* August/September 2005. http://www.motherearthnews.com/DIY/2005-08-01/The-Good-Egg.aspx

[78] Lawrence J. Appel, M.D., M.P.H. et al, "A Clinical Trial of the Effects of Dietary Patterns on Blood Pressure". *N Engl J Med* 1997; 336:1117-1124

[79] Yang, YX; Lewis JD, Epstein S, Metz DC (Dec 27 2006). "Long-term proton pump inhibitor therapy and risk of hip fracture". *Journal of the American Medical Association* 296 (24): 2947–53.

[80] RATH/PAULING U.S. PATENT # 5278189

[81] Pauling L: "Case report: Lysine/ ascorbate-related amelioration of angina pectoris". *Journal of Orthomolecular Medicine* 1991; 6: 144-146

[82] McBeath M and Pauling L: "A Case History: Lysine / Ascorbate Related Amelioration of Angina Pectoris". *J Orthomolecular Med.* 8: 1-2, 1993

[83] Pauling L: "Third case Report on Lysine / Ascorbate Amelioration of Angina Pectoris". *J. Orthomolecular Med.* 1993; (8)3: 137-138

[84] Rath M, et al. "Nutritional Supplement program halts progression of early coronary atherosclerosis documented by Ultrafast computed topography". *J Applied Nutr.* 1 9 9 6 ; 48 (3): 67-78.

[85] Duffy SJ, Gokce N, Holbrook M, et al. "Treatment of hypertension with ascorbic acid". *Lancet.* 1999;354(9195):2048-2049

[86] Harwood HJ et al. "Inhibition of human leukocyte 3-hydroxy-3-methylglutaryl coenzyme A reductase activity by ascorbic acid. An effect mediated by the free radical monodehydroascorbate". *The Journal of Biological Chemistry,* June 5, 1986: 261, 7127-7135

[87] Joel A. Simon, MD, MPH; Esther S. Hudes, PhD, MPH, "Serum Ascorbic Acid and Gallbladder Disease Prevalence Among US Adults". *Arch Intern Med*. 2000;160:931-936.

[88] Afkhami-Ardekani M Shojaoddiny-Ardekani A. "Effect of vitamin C on blood glucose, serum lipids & serum insulin in type 2 diabetes patients". *Indian J Med Res*. 2007 Nov;126(5):471-4.

[89] Enstrom JE, Kanim LE, Klein MA. "Vitamin C intake and mortality among a sample of the United States population". *Epidemiology*. 1992;3(3):194-202.

[90] Tetsuji Yokoyama, MD; Chigusa Date, PhD; Yoshihiro Kokubo, MD; Nobuo Yoshiike, MD; Yasuhiro Matsumura, PhD; Heizo Tanaka, MD, "Serum Vitamin C Concentration Was Inversely Associated With Subsequent 20-Year Incidence of Stroke in a Japanese Rural Community". *Stroke*. 2000 Oct; 31(10):2287-94.

[91] Curhan CG et al.: "A prospective study of the intake of vitamin C and B6 and the risk of kidney stones in men". *J Urol*, 1996, 155: 1847-51.

[92] Sowers MR et al.: "Prevalence of renal stones in a population-based study with dietary calcium, oxalate and medication exposures". *Am J Epidemiol*, 1998, 147: 914-20.

[93] Simon Ja, Hudes ES: "Relation of serum ascorbic acid to serum B12, serum ferritin, and kidney stones in US adults". *Arch Intern Med*,1999, 159:619-24.

[94] Curhan GC, et al.: "Intake of vitamins B6 and C and the risk of kidney stones in women". *J Am Soc Nephrol*, 1999, 10: 840-5.

[95] S. Lee et al. "Effects of oral magnesium supplementation on insulin sensitivity and blood pressure in normo-magnesemic nondiabetic overweight Korean adults". *Nutrition, Metabolism and Cardiovascular Diseases* April 2009

[96] H Teragawa, M Kato, T Yamagata, H Matsuura, G Kajiyama. "Magnesium causes nitric oxide independent coronary artery vasodilation in humans". *Heart* 2001;86:212-216

[97] Andrea Rosanoff, PhD and Mildred S. Seelig, MD. "Comparison of Mechanism and Functional Effects of Magnesium and Statin

Pharmaceuticals". *Journal of the American College of Nutrition*, Vol. 23, No. 5, 501S-505S (2004)

[98] Sarabjeet Singh et al. "Impact of subclinical thyroid disorders on coronary heart disease, cardiovascular and all-cause mortality: A meta-analysis". *International Journal of Cardiology*, March 2008; Vol 125, Issue 1: 41-48

[99] Food and Nutrition Board, Institute of Medicine. Potassium. Dietary Reference Intakes for Water, Potassium, Sodium, Chloride, and Sulfate. Washington, D. C.: National Academies Press; 2005:186-268. (National Academies Press)

[100] Singh RB, Wander GS, Rastogi A, et al. "Randomized double-blind placebo-controlled trial of coenzyme Q10 in patients with acute myocardial infarction". *Cardiovasc Drugs Ther* 1998;12:347–53.

[101] Singh RB, Neki NS, Kartikey K, et al. "Effect of coenzyme Q10 on risk of atherosclerosis in patients with recent myocardial infarction". *Mol Cell Biochem* 2003;246:75–82.

[102] Singh RB, Wander GS, Rastogi A, et al. "Randomized double-blind placebo-controlled trial of coenzyme Q10 in patients with acute myocardial infarction". *Cardiovasc Drugs Ther* 1998;12:347–53.

[103] Singh RB, Neki NS, Kartikey K, et al. "Effect of coenzyme Q10 on risk of atherosclerosis in patients with recent myocardial infarction". *Mol Cell Biochem* 2003;246:75–82.

[104] RATH/PAULING U.S. PATENT # 5278189

[105] Stampfer MJ, Hennekens CH, Manson JE, Colditz GA, Rosner B, Willett WC. "Vitamin E consumption and the risk of coronary disease in women". *N Engl J Med.* 1993 May 20;328(20):1444-9.

[106] Rimm EB, Stampfer MJ, Ascherio A, Giovannucci E, Colditz GA, Willett WC. "Vitamin E consumption and the risk of coronary heart disease in men". *N Engl J Med.* 1993 May 20;328(20):1450-6.

[107] R R Huxley and H A W Nei. "The relation between dietary flavonold intake and coronary heart disease mortality: a meta-analysis of prospective cohort studies". *European Journal of Clinical Nutrition* (2003) 57, 904–908

[108] Allen J. Taylor, M.D et al. "Extended-Release Niacin or Ezetimibe and Carotid Intima–Media Thickness. Extended-Release Niacin or

Ezetimibe and Carotid Intima—Media Thickness". *N Engl J Med* 2009; 361:2113-2122

[109] Hackam DG, Peterson JC, Spence JD. "What level of plasma homocysteine should be treated?" *Am J Hypertens* 2000;13:105–10

[110] Wang TJ, Pencina MJ, Booth SL, et al. "Vitamin D deficiency and risk of cardiovascular disease". *Circulation* 2008

[111] Pilz S, Tomaschitz A. "Role of vitamin D in arterial hypertension". *Expert Rev Cardiovasc Ther.* 2010 Nov;8(11):1599-608

[112] Appel LJ, Moore TJ, Obarzanek E, et al. "A clinical trial of the effects of dietary patterns on blood pressure". DASH Collaborative Research Group. *N Engl J Med.* 1997;336(16):1117-1124

[113] Miller GD, DiRienzo DD, Reusser ME, McCarron DA. "Benefits of dairy product consumption on blood pressure in humans: a summary of the biomedical literature". *J Am Coll Nutr.* 2000;19(2 Suppl):147S-164S.

[114] Adams J, Pepping J. "Vitamin K in the treatment and prevention of osteoporosis and arterial calcification", *Am J Health Sys Pharm*, Aug 1, 2005, vol. 62, no. 15, pp. 1574-81.

[115] Schurge crs LJ, Dissel PE, Spronk HM, et al. "Role of vitamin K and vitamin K-dependent proteins in vascular calcification". *Z Kardiol.* 2001;90 Suppl 3:57-63

[116] Benjamin B.Albert et al. "Oxidation of Marine omega-3 Supplements and Human Health". *Biomed Research International*, volume 2103 (2013).

[117] Dr. Ray Peat. "The Great Fish Oil Experiment". Retrieved on Nov 25 2012 from www.raypeat.com, http://raypeat.com/articles/articles/fishoil.shtml

[118] Stephan Guyenet. A practical Approach to Omega Fats. Whole Health Source, Ancestral Nutrition and Health. http://wholehealthsource.blogspot.ca/2008/09/pracical-approach-to-omega-fats.html., Sept 8, 2008, date of retrievalJune 12 2013

[119] Stephan Guyenet. "For Those Not Scientifically Inclined". Whole Health source, Ancestral Nutrition and Health. http://wholehealthsource.blogspot.ca/2009/05/for-those-not-

scientifically-inclined.html, May 31 2009, date of retrieval June 12, 2013

[120] *Circulation*. 2003;107:e2-e5

[121] Kim E. Innes, MSPH, PhD, Cheryl Bourguignon, RN, PhD, Ann Gill Taylor, MS, EdD. *J Am Board Fam Med*. 2005;18(6):491-519

[122] "Tai chi eases several medical conditions, reports Harvard Women's Health Watch". Harvard Health Publications, Harvard Medical School. May 2009. Dec 30 2012.Http://www.health.harvard.edu/press_releases/Tai-chi-eases-several-medical-conditions

[123] Alcohol and Heart Disease. American Heart Association Dec 30 2012. http://www.heart.org/HEARTORG/Conditions/More/MyHeartandStrokeNews/Alcohol-and-Heart-Disease_UCM_305173_Article.jsp

[124] Ornish dean et al. Can lifestyle changes reverse coronary heart disease? Volume 336, Issue 8708, Pages 129 - 133, 21 July 1990

[125] *What Your Cholesterol Levels Mean, Your Triglyceride Levels*. American Heart Association. Web. 07 June 2011. <http://www.heart.org/HEARTORG/Conditions/Cholesterol/AboutCholesterol/What-Your-Cholesterol-Levels-Mean_UCM_305562_Article.jsp>.

[126] Pyorala K. 1979 "Relationship of glucose tolerance and plasma insulin to the incidence of coronary heart disease: results from two population studies in Finland". *Diabetes Care*. 2:131–141.

[127] Welborn TA, Wearne K. *1979* "Coronary heart disease incidence and cardiovascular mortality in Busselton with reference to glucose and insulin concentrations." *Diabetes Care. 2:154–160*

[128] Ducimentiere P, Eschwege E, Papoz L, Richard JL, Claude JR, Rosselin G. 1980. "Relationship of plasma insulin level to the incidence of myocardial infarction and coronary heart disease". *Diabetologia. 19:205–210*

[129] Fontbonne A, Charles MA, Thibult N, Richard JL, Claude JR, Warnet JM, Rosselin GE, Eschwége E. 1991 "Hyperinsulinemia as a predictor of coronary heart disease mortality in a healthy

population: the Paris Prospective Study, 15-year follow-up." *Diabetologia. 34:356–361.*

[130] Matthias Rath M.D. and Linus Pauling Ph.D. "Unified Theory of Human Cardiovascular Disease Leading the Way to the Abolition of this Disease as a Cause for Human Mortality." *Journal of Orthomolecular Medicine 6: 139-143*

[131] "Risk for Ischemic Heart Disease and All-Cause Mortality in Subclinical Hypothyroidism." *The Journal of Clinical Endocrinology & Metabolism* Vol. 89, No. 7 3365-3370

[132] Vijay Nambi, MD et al. "Carotid Intima-Media Thickness and Presence or Absence of Plaque Improves Prediction of Coronary Heart Disease Risk". *J Am Coll Cardiol*, 2010; 55:1600-1607

[133] Dugald Seely et al. "Naturopathic Medicine for the Prevention of Cardiovascular Disease: a randomized clinical trial". *CMAJ*, April 292013. , doi: 10.1503/cmaj.120567

Made in the USA
Las Vegas, NV
22 January 2024

84736970R00095